PRAISE FOR NEW HORIZONS

At first glance, this book seems like it is either pure fiction or the most incredible science fiction novel of all time.

However, the inspiring stories from the patients, doctors and pharmacists mirrored my own LDN experience of pain relief in less than 48 hours. And this was after more than 35 years of disabling chronic pain.

This book is clearly destined to be a bestselling "Feel Good Book of the Year"!

It not only belongs on every bookshelf, but it should also be on every coffee table to raise awareness. And it will make a special gift to countless recipients who deserve to enjoy living again.

The LDN information and detailed case histories will educate and bring awareness to the medical community. LDN is an inexpensive drug with transitory side effects, if any.

Not since the invention of Penicillin has a drug made such a global impact. It seems almost negligent for a doctor not to prescribe LDN as it will continue to improve the lives of millions.

With long COVID continuing to dash the hopes and dreams of so many, various cancers rapidly rising in the younger population and the ongoing opioid crisis, LDN is bringing much needed hope to the World.

Linda Elsegood, the founder of LDN Research Trust has given us a "playbook" for what seems to be a miraculous pleiotropic drug. I consider this book a labor of love recounting her tireless efforts over the past 20 years.

Thank you, Linda, for giving us all "New Horizons".

Belita Anatalio, MD

This book of LDN testimonials mirrors the many positive remarks we hear also regarding daily life improvement experiences. This book is inspirational and is a must read for anyone suffering from a chronic condition. We hope more prescribers will be open to the opportunity LDN may offer those seeking help.

Eddie DeCaria, RPh, FAPC
Porter's Pharmacy and Compounding Lab

"New Horizons" is an extremely informative book and a great addition to our bookshelf. As someone who has been prescribing LDN for years, I'm always amazed at how wonderful the results can be for patients who have very limited options, if any, for treatment to improve their symptomatology and often prognosis.

Dr. Veronica A McBurnie
Clinical Director, Westbourne Medical Studios.

I would have never thought a testimonial book would prove to be such a great clinical resource for me, even though I have prescribed LDN for years. The experience my colleagues have shared here is invaluable to me and my clients.

Dr. Cheryl Winter, DCN, FNP-BC, APRN, RDN
VITAL Health Solutions

Reading testimonial after testimonial only reinforces what we do for our patients daily. We are dispensing hope. New Horizons is the perfect name, giving hope to patients suffering from many illnesses.

Steve Irsfeld RPh
Irsfeld Pharmacy

What better way to understand the potential of LDN than through the testimonials in the New Horizons book! With research progressing so quickly and across such a wide variety of conditions, this collection of experiences from prescribers, researchers, pharmacists, and patients is an excellent reference for what is possible with LDN therapies today!

Brad White RPh.
President at Medicine Center Pharmacy

For everyone who is looking for answers to health issues.

ISBN: 978-1-7391070-4-8

Published by LDN Research Trust
PO Box 1083
Buxton
Norwich
NR10 5WY
UK

www.ldnresearchtrust.org

CONTENTS

PREFACE

LDN, where to begin? Ever since the phone rang one day and a local doctor asked if we could make this new thing called "low dose naltrexone" for an MS patient, I have been hooked.

Having worked with LDN and many patients and doctors for nearly 20 years, I can absolutely and categorically say it works. It works in so many patients where nothing else has worked, and it works in diseases without standard treatments.

As a standard "allopathic" pharmacist trained in traditional medicine, I started out very sceptical - if it hadn't been for the calibre of the doctor who wanted to try LDN in his MS patient, I probably would have said no! I think about that moment often, standing in the back shop of a very dated pharmacy with a mortar and pestle and some quickly-obtained ingredients - following a formula from the 1980s, thinking... there's no way this will be a thing!

When we first started using LDN, we had very little idea of how it actually treated so many of the conditions it was being used for - it is so good to be in a place where research has caught up with clinical practice. We now have a molecular understanding of the drug effects in low doses, and a vast patient group is doing incredibly well on this novel therapy.

Getting involved in LDN is honestly one of the best decisions of my life. The road has been extremely bumpy over the years - regulatory problems, sceptical doctors and pharmacists, challenging patients with complex needs, supply chain problems - to name a few of the bumps. In our dispensary, we have a tongue-in-cheek slogan, "curing the incurable since 2006" - which probably tells you the astounding things we have seen in patients taking LDN over the years.

I look forward to continuing to work in this field for a long time to come, and I am grateful every day to the people (such as the LDN Research Trust) who have made it possible for so many people to get well when there was no other option available to them.

Stephen Dickson, MRPharmS

FOREWORD

Since my formal involvement with the LDN Research Trust in 2017, my colleagues and I that have researched naltrexone have been in awe as our knowledge base for this compound has exploded. As necessity is the motherhood of invention, when the pandemic took hold, we realized the need to repurpose old drugs (what I call hard pharma), and botanicals, herbs, vitamins and more (soft pharma) to help our patients. What we realized was that naltrexone all along was a profoundly special tool to support acute and chronic infections, autoimmunity, inflammation, and the interplay between our microbiome and our immune system.

My fascination with naltrexone has only deepened over the last (nearly) decade, since I was prescribed the original Bihari protocol (1.5 mg working up to 4.5 mg nightly) for a postpartum Hashimoto's thyroiditis flare. When people ask me why I volunteer to teach and write about LDN, I tell them that I can't get enough learning about it, on many levels and in many iterations. As a patient (I marvel at how much it reduced my chronic pain and supported my mental health, and stabilized my autoimmunity), microbiologist/immunologist (we are continuously learning about how naltrexone interacts with toll-like receptors - a key to how pathogens target our immune system), and clinician (how many of my patients have been helped by LDN).

LDN has pleiotropic effects. In pharmacology, pleiotropy includes all the drug's actions other than those for which it was specifically developed. In this case, we are constantly discovering new actions of LDN. At the 2023 international conference, we met for the first time in person since prior to the pandemic. The consensus is among the clinicians, researchers, pharmacists, and patients, that we are scratching the surface of the myriad uses for LDN, and the effective dosing regimens for different conditions.

In writing the LDN Research Trust's guides, authoring and co-authoring book chapters, speaking, and teaching, I have been thankful to reach so many people. But, by far, the most gratifying experience has been to see that patients have presented these guidelines to their clinicians, who have then prescribed LDN to them. This way, my work and the work of my colleagues will reach innumerable individuals more than I could otherwise reach on a daily basis, and will leave a legacy. Our goal remains to fund larger powered research studies and ensure patient access to a low-cost, low-risk, life-saving therapeutic agent. The credit goes to the Trust's founder, Linda Elsegood and all who volunteer tirelessly on this project.

Sarah J. Zielsdorf, MD, MS

WHAT IS LOW DOSE NALTREXONE (LDN)?

Naltrexone is a class of drug known as an opiate antagonist. It is commonly used to treat addiction to opiate drugs like heroin and morphine or to treat an acute overdose. The dosage usually varies between 50 mg to 300 mg daily, depending on the severity of the addiction. Low dose naltrexone (LDN) has been used since 1985, by Harvard-trained Dr. Bernard Bihari, a qualified neurologist from New York, USA who devised and developed the use of LDN. Dr. Bihari was qualified in internal medicine and psychiatry. We continue his pioneering work and honor his legacy.

LDN is used for chronic pain, chronic fatigue, multiple sclerosis, CFS/ME, chronic viral conditions (including COVID, long COVID and other post-viral syndromes), mast cell activation syndrome (MCAS), autoimmune diseases, and various cancers. Many autoimmune disorders respond well to LDN, and with a wide range of diseases, many clinicians will find it difficult to understand how one drug can positively affect all these pathologies. Naltrexone is an example of a drug that exhibits pleiotropy - there are many effects of this compound other than those for which the agent was specifically developed.

The first thing to understand is that naltrexone - the drug in LDN - comes in a 50:50 mixture of two different shapes (called isomers). It has been discovered that one particular shape binds to immune cells whilst the other shape binds to opioid receptors. Although consisting of exactly the same components, the two isomers appear to have different biological activity. The LEVO (left-handed) version of naltrexone blocks opiate receptors. The DEXTRO (right-handed) version blocks receptors on immune cells. These include "toll-like receptors" (TLRs), which are heavily involved in immunity. LDN is an antagonist of TLR-4. LDN has immunomodulatory, opiate blocking, and anti-tumor effects, and multiple Phase I and II trials have shown efficacy.

- "Ultra-low dose" when given daily in microgram dosing – dosed twice daily
- "Very-low dose" when given in a daily dose of less than 0.1-0.5 mg
- "Low dose" when given in daily dose (or split doses) less than or equal to 4.5-10 mg
- "Moderate dose" when the daily dose is between 10-25 mg
- "High dose" when given in daily amounts of 50 mg or more

The LDN Patient, Prescriber and Dosing Protocol Guides can be found on the website www.ldnresearchtrust.org, which are free to download. The website also contains clinical trial abstracts, conditions LDN could treat, past conference presentation videos, and much more.

Disclaimer: The information in this book does not replace medical advice. Before commencing any medical intervention, including ingestion of low dose naltrexone, it is recommended to consult with your GP and/or other medical personnel.

MEDICAL PROFESSIONALS

Erin Panian, PharmD, USA

I have been working with LDN for over 17 years. In that time, it has grown exponentially in use because more practitioners and patients are recognizing the potential benefits it can have.

Most of the time we see patients taking 1-4.5 mg for a myriad of conditions, such as GI issues, autoimmune disorders, MCAS, fertility, pain, etc. Not everyone will benefit, but we see a big enough percentage of patients benefit - and benefit greatly enough - to always think that it's worth a shot!

It is generally well tolerated and not expensive - if it doesn't work, you're not out much and if it does work it could be life changing. I have had many patients over the years tell me how it has greatly improved their life.

Angus Dalgleish, MD, FRCP, FRACP, UK

As a medical oncologist I had never heard of LDN from any professional source until I asked a patient with stage 4 cancer, who should have progressed (as we had no other active treatment available at that time), if she was taking something I did not know about. This is when I heard about LDN.

Having seen other patients who seemed to have prolonged stable disease following LDN induction I started to research its mechanisms of action. I could not attribute all the benefits to the classical opioid receptor modulation theory which was prevalent and hence looked for alternative explanations.

It was then we found that LDN blocked the inflammatory receptor that produced IL-6, or cancer growth factor as it was known.

Other unexpected activities followed and I began to realise that LDN was a supreme immune modulator with many properties of lenalidomide which I had developed with Celgene and was the first clinician to give to a human with myeloma. It is now one of the best-selling drugs in oncology. LDN has the potential to be far more successful as it is active in even more cancers and other chronic inflammatory and autoimmune conditions.

Shellie Skala, Pharmacy Technician III, USA

Our pharmacy first learned of LDN in early 2019 at the inquiry of a patient. We began researching LDN, viewed webinars and learned how to compound it. By late spring of 2019, we had our first patients using LDN.

We have compounded LDN to successfully treat a multitude of conditions, including chronic pain, fibromyalgia, anxiety, psoriasis, and RSD. Many of our patients have been on LDN for several years and report vast improvements in quality of life. Our patients also appreciate having an effective treatment that is low-cost.

One memorable patient was Richard. He was a 68-year-old man when he came in with a prescription for LDN 1.5 mg to treat his chronic back pain. After about three months he increased to 3 mg. He felt a great amount of relief and has stayed at that dose for three years. He is now back to doing his regular daily activities.

Nasha Winters, ND, FABNO, USA

As noted in my chapter in the third LDN book, I had the distinct pleasure of meeting and learning under Dr. Bihari while working in a HIV/AIDS clinic in Arizona in the mid 1990s. First-hand experience with the guru himself for which I am immensely grateful.

Later, my practice evolved into using LDN in autoimmune conditions and cancer. Today, LDN continues to be a staple in my integrative oncology consulting practice where I get to educate physicians all over the world on the best ways to support their patients based on my methodology of Test, Assess, Address, Never Guess. (™)

It has become increasingly helpful in tandem with the standard of care immune therapies being offered in which LDN seems to enhance their effect while protecting the often-incapacitating autoimmune side effects these drugs can elicit.

And personally, this is a therapy I have used to support my own terrain while addressing all of my previous autoimmune patterns including RA, Hashimoto's, celiac, PCOS and endometriosis - a game changer for sure.

Amalia Fantasia, PhD, "Dr. Molly," USA

LDN is as close to Holy Water as you can get. In conjunction with the use of proper nutraceuticals, we have seen remarkable results or recoveries in so many of our patients. Utilizing it in our facility has been one of the best implementations to our care protocols that we have done.

We routinely prescribe an LDN tincture for those with cancer, post-Lyme or chronic Lyme disease, pain syndromes, long COVID, neurological diseases, gastrointestinal disorders and more. The liquid form of LDN is particularly valuable for those with GI issues, as other methods of dosing may not have benefited them well enough otherwise.

We have seen significant improvements in levels of pain, inflammation, and fatigue across the board - ultimately improving our patients' overall quality of life. I am so glad to see that more and more practitioners are finally recognizing the benefits that LDN can have for their many patients

CJ McCarrick, FRACGP, Australia

I first became aware of the potential therapeutic benefit of LDN about two years ago. Having learned more about it, it is an exciting therapeutic option to potentially benefit patients with conditions that are difficult to manage, such as chronic fatigue syndrome and fibromyalgia.

Generally side effects are mild, such as insomnia or gastric upset, but tend to be avoided with a very slow titration process. Several patients have reported improvements in their symptoms and I consider it worth trialling in such patients where standard therapies have not been successful. I find it even more effective in combination with a ketogenic diet, when trying to improve autoimmune conditions.

Stefanie Werner, NMD, USA

LDN has proven to be a versatile and effective tool when I tackle a variety of chronic conditions such as autoimmune disorders, pain, infection, inflammatory conditions, and even certain neurological diseases. LDN provides a unique mechanism of action, highlighting its ability to modulate both the immune and endorphin system, making this an excellent resource for both medical professionals and patients seeking to improve therapeutic outcomes and gain results.

Akila Dungarwalla, Pharmacist Independent Prescriber, UK

I first began prescribing LDN in 2022 after hearing about it from the LDN Research Trust. Since then, I have been prescribing LDN as a successful form of treatment for a variety of patients who suffer from various autoimmune diseases including fibromyalgia, MS, ME, chronic fatigue syndrome, rheumatoid arthritis, hyperthyroidism and more recently, long COVID.

I start my patients on an initial dose of 0.5 mg to 1 mg and gradually increase the dosage on a case-by-case basis. Currently, the highest dose I have prescribed to a patient is 4.5 mg. Since beginning my LDN prescriber journey I have not had any patients report that they have experienced no effect, and at least 60-70% have reported the benefits. In addition, I have had very minimal reports of side effects and usually swapping my patients to a morning dose sees these subside.

The most important improvement I see in my LDN patients is the return of their "buzz." They experience an increase in energy, their brain fog lifts, they feel strong enough to perform daily tasks and they have a sense of relief knowing that something is working - feelings that many of my patients have not experienced for years.

As stated above, many of my patients experience the great benefits of LDN, but a few specific cases come to mind when looking at the life-changing impact this treatment has.

Lisa first started experiencing severe back pain during the spring of 2020, and was subsequently diagnosed with secondary breast cancer, with extensive bone metastases, in autumn that year. By then she had been in severe pain for several months and was left feeling exhausted from the lack of sleep and the constant agony. She had been offered morphine for the pain, but made the decision that she did not want to resort to this on a long-term basis. After being made aware of LDN through the CancerActive website, she decided to give it a go, as following diagnosis, her symptoms have partially but not fully been resolved by radiotherapy. Currently, she is not experiencing any side effects, is able to sleep, has found great relief in her pain, and strongly believes that LDN has benefitted her immune system - as she has already outlived her original prognosis.

As mentioned before, many of my long COVID patients have found that LDN has allowed them to return to living as opposed to simply surviving. Isolda began experiencing symptoms following a COVID infection in January 2022: her life got gradually worse, she described it as almost unmanageable for a good few months. She was constantly slightly out of breath, unable to walk for more than 5-10 minutes because of POTS, ME/CFS, dysautonomia, experienced extremely bad sleep due to the onset of sleep apnoea, and presented with wild fluctuation of oxygen levels during the day as well, desaturation down to 85% at times.

After countless visits to many doctors, where she was offered nothing as a result of the lack of protocol for the treatment of long COVID, she went searching for avenues to individually treat each of her symptoms. LDN came to her attention in the context of ME/CFS and then shortly thereafter through studies commissioned specifically for long COVID. As a bonus she discovered how LDN can be beneficial to a wider set of autoimmune diseases that she had been previously diagnosed with. And so her LDN journey began! She experienced definitive improvements from day one, getting her first good night's sleep in months. Gradually all her symptoms began to wane and after a year and a half, she is able to work full days and begin building her fitness!

This treatment breathes life back into patients who have suffered with no relief for far too long. It is my hope that the benefits of LDN are further researched and shared with the wider public. We will continue to support our patients with LDN.

Pamela W. Smith, MD, MPH, MS, USA

There have been two things that have really changed medicine in my 46 years of practice. No, it is not CT scan, MRI, or ultrasound, all of which came about starting when I was in medical school. One of those two is low dose naltrexone. The other is bio-identical hormones. Almost every disease process is inflammatory in nature. Both LDN and bio-identical hormones are anti-inflammatory.

Most of my practice, including myself and my husband, are on LDN. It really has been a godsend to myself, family, friends, and patients.

Ronal Perino, MD, Brazil

I first heard about LDN when I was on a course taught by a Brazilian doctor called Lair Ribeiro. I first prescribed it for a patient about six months ago. I start with a dose of 3 mg and ask the patient to increase to 4.5 mg if needed. I would say that perhaps 70% of my patients receive benefits from taking LDN, as evidenced in the improvement in the patients' conditions. Some brief case studies are as follows:

Case One: I had a patient who used Remicade, a chimeric monoclonal antibody for ankylosing spondylitis, an autoimmune disease. In Brazil this medication is given to the patient free of charge by our health system. I explained to him to use LDN too because I thought it would have more benefits, it would be better for him. So he started using LDN. Our health system failed to provide Remicade for two months but he didn't miss it at all, the LDN was enough, he was no longer in pain, he did not miss the Remicade.

Case Two: I had a patient with corneal ocular pain. She had had cataract surgery three years earlier but she still had a lot of eye pain. She visited several doctors and used different medications such as lubricants, pain killers, eye drops of all kinds and medicines for allergies, dry eyes and inflammation, but nothing resolved her pain during those three years. She came to my clinic for a consultation, I decided to prescribe LDN for her. Within two weeks, she had no more eye pain.

Angie Fielden, LDN Specialist, USA

My quality of life is back, and I'm pain free. During the height of COVID-19, specifically in August 2020, my husband, my sister, and I started taking LDN. We did this mainly for the extra protection against the devastation COVID might cause anyone of us. I had attended several LDN conferences during 2020 and I became more aware of LDN's abilities to help with the effects caused by COVID-19, particularly after I'd listened to a pharmacist by the name of Sebastian Denison.

His lecture was so good, it was on post-COVID-19 treatment options and LDN. At that point, I knew this could possibly save my sister, husband, or my own life should we contract COVID-19. There was a bit of fear within our family as we had already lost two members of our family and almost a third family member to COVID-19. One that passed away was fully vaccinated and boosted, and two were not, and the two that passed away were very healthy otherwise. This is why we decided to begin LDN.

I didn't realize the benefits that would come soon after beginning LDN therapy. I heard in other LDN lectures that LDN binds to the toll-like receptor 4. Therefore, one could say it acts as an immunomodulator as well as lowering the inflammation in the body. For those reasons, all three of us, my husband, my sister, and I started on LDN. Shortly after we all reported having less joint pain. My sister and I suffer from arthritis in our hands and other places throughout our bodies, while my husband has some neuropathy and joint pain, mainly in his knees.

Within about two weeks, I noticed I was sleeping much better. My thumbs and hip pain used to be so excruciating at night I would flip-flop about every 30 minutes. It seemed as if I would never get a good night's sleep, and I remembered being so tired all the time as well as foggy thinking. I would get up and walk around or go to the restroom several times a night to get a little relief. Now, I sleep mostly through the night, and five out of seven nights, I only get out of bed once my alarm goes off. I also could not do many things I love, like riding my motorcycle or working out with weights, which I used to enjoy but had to stop because of hand or hip pain. Now, just like being able to sleep at night again, my husband and I can ride our motorcycles for hours at a time. In addition, I work out three days a week with weights. My grip is better, and I am not in pain anymore.

My sister believes in her heart that LDN saved her life. She got COVID-19 around the same time we lost one of our family members. With her having several comorbidities, she and I felt she was at high risk for mortality if she contracted COVID-19. Our worst nightmare happened just four and a half months after beginning LDN, and she contracted COVID-19. Before you panic, she is still very much alive and doing great. Not only did she make it through COVID-19, but she also was never hospitalized or placed on any medications while having COVID-19. Within six to seven days, she was almost back to normal other than being a little tired. She also has a reduction of arthritis pain since taking LDN daily.

I believe in LDN, so much so that I took the masterclass course with the LDN Research Trust to become an LDN Specialist. This is a great benefit for the compounding pharmacy I work for. It has helped me to speak with providers and patients about LDN's benefits with many disease states. Being a patient first and seeing my results gave me the passion and drive I needed to help others achieve what I have found. As a result, my quality of life is back, and I am pain free.

Lori Allen, RPh, USA

I have been compounding LDN since 2004 and have worked with thousands of physicians and patients through the years. It is so rewarding when a patient responds to LDN and is able to gain their health and lives back. I am always very leery of something that touches so many health conditions, but this is the real deal. While it doesn't work for everyone, it works so frequently that it is one of my most-compounded prescriptions. I work with hundreds of patients, dispensing thousands of doses each month.

One of my favorite LDN stories is of a patient who was a life coach. She came to me so exhausted that she wasn't working, couldn't keep up with her home and her husband was scared for her. She started on the 1.5 mg dose and called me after her first dose asking if this was legal because she hadn't had this kind of clarity or energy in years. I assured her that it was completely legal and I was so happy that she was responding so positively.

She then called back a couple of days later because her sleep was disrupted. We worked on lowering her dose because she is one of my super-sensitive patients. She gradually worked up the dose as her body allowed and was able to function again. She continued for a year with LDN and then decided she wanted to try going off the LDN because she preferred to let her body work on its own. She lasted about a month before her husband begged her to go back on LDN as they saw the drastic decline in her health, mental status and energy. Once she had resumed LDN she continued to thrive and live life to the fullest. This is one of my superstar stories.

The great majority of patients do not have this dramatic of a response, but most do find benefit from adding LDN to their daily routine. They find the inflammation decreases and mental wellbeing increases which translates to a positive outcome. Some don't realize the impact the LDN has until they stop taking the medication and then they realize how much the LDN has reduced their symptoms.

I hope you will find a practitioner or are a practitioner who is open minded to working with a medication that has proven itself safe and effective when being used for a purpose other than its original development and indication. Because naltrexone has been around for so long, there isn't incentive for a large pharmaceutical company to invest in the expense to gain the green light from the FDA for another indication.

The community that surrounds the LDN Research Trust has gained so much empirical evidence through use and discussion with other practitioners, pharmacists and patients and continues to expand the practical use of LDN for various conditions. I wish you the best in your journey with LDN!

Dagmara Beine, PA-C, PhD, USA

With over five years of experience prescribing LDN in my practice I have witnessed its impact on a wide spectrum of conditions, leading me to consider it one of my favorite therapies in the field.

LDN's versatility shines through its off-label applications, garnering attention from practitioners worldwide for its efficacy in diverse disease types such as autoimmune disorders, multiple sclerosis, pain management, and cancer treatment. LDN has demonstrated its potential to intercept cell signaling pathways, modify immune responses, and impede tumor growth. I have also seen great success using LDN for anxiety and depression, and even in cases of extreme inflammation.

One of LDN's remarkable attributes that is highly relevant to many of my patients is its ability to synergize with traditional anticancer therapies like radiation and platinum chemotherapy drugs.

In summary, I have seen LDN be the missing piece for many of my patients, and I feel grateful to have this tool available to us.

Christine Salter, MD, DC, USA

I first heard about low dose naltrexone (LDN) around 14 years ago. A potential patient with Hashimoto's thyroiditis asked if I would prescribe it. Since I had only heard of naltrexone in the context of opioid overdose, I felt that I should do my due diligence regarding the low dose uses before I responded to her request. I was intrigued with Dr. Bihari's work with patients who were diagnosed with HIV, and his subsequent work with patients diagnosed with autoimmune disease.

I started to prescribe LDN for autoimmunity and then for patients diagnosed with cancer, after attending a conference in Chicago. I heard several presentations on LDN including one in particular where it was used along with alpha-lipoic acid for pancreatic cancer.

Over the past several years, I have seen excellent responses in my patients with autoimmune conditions such as Hashimoto's thyroiditis, rheumatoid arthritis and non-specific autoimmunity. In addition, LDN is foundational in my integrative oncology practice.

Cliff Holt, RPh, USA

I remember sitting in a PCCA meeting in Chicago and one of the speakers was Linda Elsegood, founder of the LDN Research Trust. She spoke about naltrexone, which had been around for decades, in a new way. The thing that still stands out to me is how passionate Linda was and her success story with LDN. She also gave many examples of indications where LDN has benefited patients.

I came home from that conference and ordered 12 LDN books to pass out to local providers. We started compounding LDN within seven days.

We now have many success stories with our own patients. LDN therapy has positively changed the lives of so many patients! And we have only touched the tip of the iceberg!

One patient that comes to mind had psoriatic arthritis. It got so bad that he could no longer work or travel. He had tried several therapies over the last five years. LDN gave him his quality of life back.

Paul Marik, MD, USA

Low dose naltrexone (LDN) has fascinating pharmacologic properties. Naltrexone is an opioid receptor antagonist that has been used for decades for opiate addiction.

It was noted that in certain patients being treated with naltrexone for an opioid addiction many reported significant secondary benefit when being weaned off naltrexone. This group of patients had chronic inflammatory and autoimmune conditions and reported improvements whilst using the lower doses of naltrexone.

LDN has therefore emerged as a useful drug for a spectrum of chronic inflammatory diseases. We strongly advocate the use of LDN for our vaccine-injured patients; in addition, there have also been recent anecdotal reports of cancer resolution following the use of LDN. In patients with cancer, LDN is usually used in combination with other agents.

Harpal Bains, MBBS, DFSRH, PGCAestMed, UK

I first came across LDN when I was researching various gut protocols for complex gut dysbiosis and came across it being mentioned in Chris Kresser's blog post. I have met Chris and appreciated his attention to detail in complex conditions. I had never heard of LDN and so decided to research it. What I read blew my mind and the simplicity of its mechanism of action simply made sense and appealed to my personal approach to complex diseases. I then found out about the LDN Research Trust which gave me more confidence in prescribing a medication I wasn't familiar with. I decided to trial it in some of my patients with autoimmune conditions, starting with multiple sclerosis and Hashimoto's thyroiditis. I didn't know what to expect but hoped that my patients would simply get a better sense of wellbeing with fewer trigger attacks, which was exactly what happened.

Since then, it has been a huge learning curve where only experience in trialling it in different conditions made sense. To date, we advise it in every autoimmune condition, every condition where low immune status may be a concern (like HIV and cancers), gut issues and even in well people who prefer being proactive about their health and choose to boost their immunity. We have found the right words to encourage use of LDN especially when patients have a hard time with side effects. A lot of this experience has been shared with other practitioners at conferences held by the LDN Research Trust which has been critical in supporting practitioners and continued learning in this niche area of medicine. If we all put our heads together and spread the word about this simple and safe drug, we will be able to help many more people. That is the ultimate hope.

Philip Giordano, RPh, USA

I first heard about LDN 20 years ago from my former partner Dr. Skip Lenz. That is when we started compounding all forms of LDN.

We followed the recommendations of Dr. Bernard Bihari and to date use the same protocols starting at 1.5 mg at bedtime working up to 4.5 mg. We have seen doses as high as 12 mg for appetite suppression.

I believe that 80% of our patients receive some benefit from the therapy. Many tests, including MRI of the spine and brain as well as antibody titers for Hashimoto's, show real improvement with prolonged therapy.

We ship all over the country, and encountered a patient with a very rare form of Lyme disease. The patient was bedridden and nearly blind as a result of neurological complications from Lyme. His doctors had given up hope on any therapies they knew of. We had suggested trying the naltrexone at 4.5 mg at bedtime. This patient not only recovered within weeks; he then was also able to drive within one month of initiating therapy! His family was so grateful that they made a trip from their home in Rochester, NY to see us and thank us personally in South Florida.

LDN has been a godsend to so many. We will continue to provide a quality product at a reasonable cost to anyone who has a valid prescription.

Gregory A. Plotnikoff, MD, MTS, FACP, USA

I first began prescribing LDN for internal medicine patients about 25 years ago after learning about LDN from my father, Nicholas Plotnikoff, PhD, a psychoneuroimmunopharmacologist studying metenkephalin. This immune modulating peptide's endogenous production appears to increase with use of LDN. He and Bernie Bihari, MD, were in close contact for years because of the potential benefit they saw for innumerable patients.

At this time, I prescribe LDN in the following situations:
- Several autoimmune conditions
- Ehlers-Danlos/hypermobility-associated pain and other chronic pain conditions
- Mast cell activation syndromes (MCAS)
- Long COVID
- Intestinal dysmotility
- Adjunctive cancer therapy including for management of aromatase inhibitor pain syndromes
- Some forms of chronic fatigue
- Some forms of immunosuppression

I am full of happy stories with LDN for each of the above categories. To illustrate the power of LDN for persons in my clinic, I share a story that is better illustrated in the following case report by Dr. Pradeep Chopra and Mark S. Cooper. This is an awesome case report on LDN and CRPS entitled "Treatment of Complex Regional Pain Syndrome (CRPS) Using Low Dose Naltrexone (LDN)" published online April 2nd 2013.

A 48-year-old male veteran, in 2006, developed the following CRPS symptoms in his right lower extremity after an injury to his right leg: swelling, allodynia (pain to normal touch), color change, temperature change, and some weakness. By 2007, the patient developed moderate CRPS symptoms in his upper extremities. In 2008, he developed blisters and skin ulceration in his right lower leg. At this time, the patient was being treated with opioids, pregabalin, and duloxetine.

By 2009, the patient's pain had become severe enough that he could not walk without assistance. In 2010, he underwent a cardiac bypass surgery for coronary artery disease. His CRPS symptoms became widespread after this surgery, spreading to his upper chest, upper arms, and forearms. In 2011, the patient developed significant dystonic spasms to both upper extremities, resulting in hyperextension of his fingers. From 2008 to 2012, the patient underwent multiple treatments with anticonvulsants, antidepressants, physical therapy, psychotherapy, topical and systemic analgesics, including but not limited to opioids.

In August of 2011 to January 2012, the patient was treated with lower dose intravenous ketamine infusions and his use of the opioid oxycodone was changed to tapentadol. This narcotic was removed for one week prior to starting low dose naltrexone, which was started and maintained at 4.5 mg per day (one dose at night). Additional medications included metformin, tramadol, valsartan, clorazepate, simvastatin, fish oil, and vitamin C.

Immediately before LDN treatment, the patient had patchy areas of allodynia of his right foot, extensive areas of dysesthesia (skin-on-fire feeling) in his right leg below the knee and heel of his foot, as well as bilaterally dysesthesia in his arms. There were significant color and temperature changes in the right foot compared to the left foot, as well as pitting edema in the right foot.

By March of 2012, the patient's requirements for the lower dose intravenous ketamine infusions were not as frequent, pain spikes not as high. The patient recovered from CRPS flares more quickly, felt more energetic, and tolerated pain better. He became physically more active, and his sleep improved significantly. Within two months after starting LDN, the patient's dystonic spasms discontinued, although he still had moderate pain in both arms. The patient was able to walk without a cane, which he had used continuously since 2006. After LDN therapy, the patient's pain symptoms have reduced in severity, but not in their distribution. His current mood state is good. No side effects of LDN were noted. The before and after photos in this case study online are unmistakably powerful.

LDN deserves much more research as a low-cost, low-toxicity, intervention with great promise. I hope each reader of this will share with others the importance of advancing knowledge on this topic among both patients and clinicians.

Ginevra Liptan, MD, USA

I have experienced the benefits of LDN for fibromyalgia on both a personal and professional level. It is one of the first treatments I add for new patients, and about two thirds report pain reduction.

I have been prescribing LDN for fibromyalgia over seven years and have learned through trial and error that there are even ways to safely use LDN in many patients that also take opioid pain medications.

Unfortunately, many health care providers are not aware of LDN, in spite of good clinical and research evidence supporting its use. That's why I go into so much detail about it in my book about fibromyalgia, which you can find online.

Trip Hoffman, PharmD, USA

I first learned about LDN around 2010 from a PCCA conference and have been compounding with LDN and promoting LDN ever since. We have compounded LDN for many different diagnoses, including, but not strictly limited to, chronic pain, chronic inflammation conditions, rheumatoid arthritis, irritable bowel syndrome (IBS), Crohn's, lupus, MS, thyroid issues (both Graves' and Hashimoto's), long COVID, depression, anxiety, weight loss, chronic pruritis/itching (topical and vaginal), and lichen planus.

We have experienced an overwhelming positive result across the board with various autoimmune conditions, both with newly diagnosed and those with a diagnosis of many years.

Another intriguing and positive response is for acral lick dermatitis in canines. We have seen great success utilizing a combination of an oral capsule (weight-based) with a topical 1% LDN in ZoSil cream by PCCA. The canine response has been remarkable and our patients (and veterinarians) are extremely thankful. We have also used LDN as an adjunctive therapy in pets (cats and dogs) to improve the quality of life and to potentially extend life for those fighting certain cancers.

Edyta Biernat-Kaluza, MD, Poland

I first heard about LDN from a patient I was treating for rheumatoid arthritis (RA). This patient was a gynaecologist.

The first patient I prescribed LDN to was a young lady suffering from RA who wanted to become pregnant. As she was taking methotrexate pregnancy wasn't advisable. After some discussion she stopped taking methotrexate and I started her on LDN at 1.5 mg for ten days, then 3 mg for a further ten days, increasing to 4.5 mg. This is the dose that she used consistently for many months. The benefits of reduced pain and oedema in her joints was very promising.

As a rheumatologist, I generally treat patients with autoimmunological diseases: rheumatoid arthritis, psoriatic arthritis, ankylosing spondylitis, systemic lupus erythematosus (SLE) and so on. In these patients I start them on, as mentioned earlier, 1.5 mg, later 3 mg and usually chronically 4.5 mg. The doses for children depend on their body mass, but generally I start with 0.1 mg. Lately, I treat adult fibromyalgia patients with a different protocol - VLDN (very low dose naltrexone) four times a day, every six hours. The highest dose I have prescribed in clinical practice was 11 mg. I see benefits in about 60% of my patients.

During LDN treatment patients generally have better mood, they report more energy, some of them report better sleep and immunity improvement. Rheumatic patients notice better quality of life, less pain, better range of movement in affected joints. I see a reduction of inflammation parameters and serological improvement (ANA, RF and so on).

I had an occasion to present the following case during an LDN conference in Nassau in 2020. A 37-year-old SLE patient with pleuritis and lupus nephritis history. In the past she was treated with cyclophosphamide plus MMF, and later she took steroids for many years. She appeared in my office in 2017 with symptoms of polyarthritis. She was informed by her nephrologist that she could not become pregnant. Her other conditions were non-alcoholic steatohepatitis (NASH) and Hashimoto's. In laboratory tests she had leukopenia, elevated fibrinogen and elevated ANA 640 and ATG. She was prescribed hydroxychloroquine and LDN treatment was started (1.5 mg; 3 mg; 4.5 mg). After six weeks of LDN therapy, for the first time in her life, she got pregnant. At 24 weeks gestation she had to be hospitalized due to amenorrhea. The pregnancy ended with premature delivery at 27 weeks. After the birth, she continued LDN and expressed breast milk. She has continued LDN therapy at her present dose of 4.5 mg (her former dose being 6 mg). Currently her baby girl is five years old and very healthy.

I personally take LDN for MS, which appeared 27 years ago after a tetanus vaccination. Six weeks after the injection I noticed right side paresis causing driving difficulties. For these years I received only two pulses of steroids, intravenous and intramuscular injections with various B vitamins. I use high doses of vitamin D3, too. I was offered interferon, but I decided not to take this treatment.

I started LDN in 2015 at 1.5 mg, later 3 mg and then 4.5 mg which I still take now. In the beginning I experienced "vivid dreams," so I chose to take LDN in the morning which solved this issue. I noticed my general condition improved after just two weeks. At present, I use LDN, vitamin D3, vitamin B, Q10, glutathione, alpha-lipoic acid and butyric acid.

Taking LDN is the only solution for me to be in very good condition.

I suffer from various immunological problems: MS, reactive arthritis, pre-myeloma condition, and LDN helps to control the symptoms of all of these - autoimmunological and hemato/oncological.

As a PhD rheumatologist with 30 years of clinical experience, I regret that treatment with LDN is only mentioned occasionally among my Polish and international colleagues in the fibromyalgia field, but not in autoimmunological diseases.

Mark W. Ernest, MD, USA

I initially came across LDN in pursuit of integrative medicine strategies to broaden the spectrum of treatment choices for my patients. I have administered it for a wide array of conditions, including but not limited to opiate use disorder, treatment resistant depression, and various neurologic disorders, all with very positive outcomes.

Its multifaceted applications make it an essential and invaluable asset in treatment, and its efficacy continues to impress.

Sajad Zalzala, MD, USA

I became interested in integrative medicine during medical school. In fact, if it were not for integrative medicine, I would have dropped out after my first year of medical school. The conventional medical approach of being reactive and treating symptoms just did not resonate with me - but integrative medicine really sparked my curiosity and passion for helping people.

As a student, I started seeking out local doctors who were practicing integrative medicine and started to learn from them, and attend conferences and read books and listen to podcasts as part of my quest to use functional and integrative medicine to help patients.

I learned about LDN during one of these integrative medicine conferences back in 2006 or 2007 and was immediately drawn to its potential as a power therapeutic. I continued to learn about LDN over the next several years until I was finally able to prescribe it to my patients starting in 2012.

Through my private clinical practice, I started out prescribing LDN to patients who had been diagnosed with fibromyalgia and chronic fatigue with very promising results. I had also read about its potential for Crohn's disease and ulcerative colitis and found that it was also very useful for many patients. Over time, I started expanding the conditions where I thought LDN would be helpful to include almost any condition with a neuropathic, inflammatory, or autoimmune component - and the list of conditions grew very quickly and is quite long. I often joke with patients that "you name the condition, and LDN can mostly likely be beneficial."

In 2016, I started getting into telemedicine and saw a need to help patients obtain prescriptions for LDN, so I launched a telemedicine service. Through this service, I have helped thousands of patients obtain prescriptions for LDN, and many of them have reported good results reducing symptoms across a wide array of diseases, conditions, and syndromes. It got to the point where people would read about LDN for their rare disease or condition, then ask me if I thought LDN would be helpful.

One example is Hailey-Hailey disease (HHD) - a condition we don't even learn in medical school and I had never heard of previously. It started with one patient, then several, asking if LDN could help. I read about the condition and it seemed to have an inflammatory component to it and I told patients that it might be worth a try if they are willing. Some patients with HHD seemed to respond to it well and were very thankful to have the opportunity to try LDN, since they really had no other treatment option. This is one example out of many conditions.

There are some people who respond wonderfully to LDN - I call them the "super-responders." In my estimation, those account for about 10 to 20% of LDN users. Most users, however, fall in the "partial responders" where they find some benefit from LDN, but it's not "life changing."

Unfortunately, not every patient responds to LDN and I wish I could figure out why. In my experience, anywhere between 50 to 70% of patients respond to LDN (the "super" and "partial" responders combined) - and success rates depends on the type of condition and other factors. Some conditions, like psoriasis, seem to have a lower response rate, whereas fibromyalgia syndrome seems to have a slightly higher response rate.

Allowing patients to self-titrate their own dose seems to help improve response rates, but I still regret that response rates remain stubborn at that 50 to 70% rate. I hope to be able to figure out one day why some people don't respond, and what we can do to get those 30 to 50% of non-responders to appreciate the wonders of LDN.

Stephan Alpiger, MD, Denmark

I have been a pain doctor for about 19 years. I began to prescribe LDN about 12 years ago. In the beginning mainly to fibromyalgia patients. I have noticed that LDN helps in about 74% of FM patients. Later I began to prescribe LDN to help other conditions like neuropathic pain, post-corona condition, whiplash syndrome, fatigue, etc.

Now we work online and have patients all over the EU including Switzerland and Norway. We collaborate with pharmacies in Germany, Holland, Denmark and Switzerland.

Burt Berkson, MD, MS, PhD, USA

I first heard about LDN from a prostate cancer patient in 1999 who told me that he was getting better on it. I started prescribing it to my cancer patients along with alpha-lipoic acid and many of them reversed their disease.

We probably have the best results with autoimmune disease, especially systemic lupus erythematosus (SLE). Many of these patients are free of their condition after only a few months just using LDN. I have found that LDN is a remarkably effective medicine for the treatment of several disease states.

Deanna Windham, DO, USA

Over the two decades of my career, low dose naltrexone (LDN) has been one of my most-used and consistently-effective treatments for many disease processes including all forms of autoimmune disease and cancer, hormonal imbalance at all ages, autism and ADHD, frequent infections and many more.

LDN has a wide range of positive impact in the microbiome,

immune system, brain, cardiovascular system and whole body, with no life threatening or even significant side effects when used by a knowledgeable physician.

I have seen hundreds of patients have dramatic improvement in even very long-term symptoms with the addition of LDN to their treatment plan. It is so beneficial in so many different disease and anti-aging processes that I consider it negligent not to consistently utilize this medication when appropriate.

Michael Vuong, RPh, USA

Before starting here at this pharmacy, I was familiar with naltrexone over the years as a commercial 50 mg tablet that has been used traditionally as a competitive opioid blocker. Since working here, I've seen low doses of naltrexone help patients with diseases associated with the autoimmune system.

I recall a patient with severe mast cell activation syndrome whose symptoms had not improved using traditional therapy. Her provider wanted her to try LDN and called in a prescription. Later on, when I called the office for refill authorization, her provider informed us that LDN was beneficial to her. The patient informed me that she was doing a lot better.

The side effect profile appears favorable for patients taking LDN. Our feedback for side effects associated with LDN typically includes vivid dreams and occasional GI disturbance which are generally transitory.

Results may vary, but the feedback provided by our patients, who suffer from all manner of autoimmune diseases, has been very positive. I am proud to be part of a team at our pharmacy that can compound LDN and make such a positive difference to the quality of life for so many people.

Jodi Peterson – Pharmacy Owner, USA

LDN has been something I have been passionate about since the early 2000s after reading an article in the *International Journal of Pharmaceutical Compounding*. As someone that worked for a compounding pharmacy, and then eventually became an owner of one myself, it seemed like inflammatory and autoimmune conditions were so prevalent no matter the practice setting.

When I would visit with providers to see what we could help them with, there was an overwhelming need to help with various conditions rooted in inflammation. After reading the article about LDN, I immediately started gathering more information to provide to the various providers we worked with. Several providers were excited to start prescribing and others were apprehensive due to the lack of information, studies and testimonials.

Today, we have an abundant number of providers that send their patients to us for LDN prescriptions. I commend the organizations/organizers of the many conferences in the last couple of years that are educating providers about the benefits of LDN. The LDN Research Trust has been an excellent resource and I am very proud to be a member. The most rewarding part of this journey has been the patients that come into the pharmacy that are taking LDN and seeing their symptoms/disease state improving and the smiles on their faces.

Paul S. Anderson, NMD, USA

As a physician whose practice is split between oncology and advanced complex illness (both pediatric and adult) patients I attempt to find and use as broad an array of therapies as possible. Low dose naltrexone (LDN) has become one of the core therapies in both my cancer and chronic illness patient populations. I have used LDN in practice for over 15 years now and find it invaluable as a clinical tool.

Through the years I have incorporated LDN into the oncology side of my practice more and more. With continual increases in scientific data supporting the use of LDN in oncology I find more places where it can support patients through standard and targeted therapies. It is truly rare in my practice to have an oncology patient not using LDN.

On the chronic illness side of my practice, I have employed LDN in my pediatric and adult autoimmune, post-infectious, and neuroinflammatory patients. These patients often find their other integrative therapies synergized by the addition of LDN.

For these past many years, I can honestly say that my practice has been enhanced by the use of LDN in all patient types.

Elliot Udell, MD, USA

I first heard about LDN from the medical literature, at least three years ago. It was then that I first started prescribing LDN for appropriate patients. I start the dosage at 2 mg per day for a week then 3 mg a day for a week and then 4.5 mg for as long as the patient needs it. I tend not to go above 4.5 mg daily.

I would say that 90% of my patients receive benefit from LDN. The results that I use to show improvement is to track on a 1-10 scale the amount of pain reduction the patient is having. For example, if a patient presents 8 on the pain scale and with LDN levels off at 6 and the patient is happy with the results, I'll continue it. There are some patients that have gone from 8 to zero but that is rare.

One interesting patient that I have treated was a 32-year-old Caucasian female who presented with erythromelalgia. Her feet were lobster red and she was in extreme pain. She was taking duloxetine 60 mg daily but was still in pain. With low dose naltrexone combined with the duloxetine she no longer has foot pain even though the redness may still be present at times. The way I know if the patient is happy with the medication is that the patient refills the meds when she runs out of them and she has no desire to discontinue either one.

I have many more cases. I lecture about these cases at medical conferences and have educated many other doctors on the benefits of LDN in appropriate cases.

Elizabeth Livengood, NMD, USA

I learned about LDN in my residency just as *The LDN Book, Volume 1* was published. We quickly applied this information in our clinic in cases of multiple sclerosis and other autoimmune conditions. I still use LDN with most of my autoimmune patients, all long-haul COVID patients and many depression patients.

Roughly 90% of my patients experience benefits with the remaining 10% having unusual side effects such as an allergic reaction or aggravated symptoms. Approximately 25 to 30% of my LDN patients will end up moving their medication to a morning dosing regimen to mitigate sleep disturbances or other similar side effects.

While I have seen biomarkers such as antibodies or sedimentation rates decline with the use of LDN, I rely more on clinical information and reduction in symptoms to monitor efficacy. For example, a patient came to me with over a decade of debilitating fibromyalgia which was affecting her quality of life severely. She could not do more than one activity per day due to exhaustion and pain. After starting LDN along with nutritional IV therapy, she experienced significant improvement in sleep, energy, mood and cognitive function; and reduced frequency and severity of migraines and joint pains. She also noted improvement in her nails and skin. She was able to reduce her number of other supplement and pharmaceutical pills taken daily from 30 to 10! More importantly she is able to get back to the activities she enjoys most such as riding horses, and reports feeling "ten years younger" since starting LDN.

Sebastian Denison, RPh, USA

It was back in 1999/2000 when I first learned about LDN as a compounding pharmacy staff member, and I started to understand its value in a patient-focused health care practice. LDN was being used in MS and fibromyalgia patients, and all of them had the same feedback on benefit and how it had minimal side effects.

We were compounding the normal standard doses (1.5-3-4.5 mg) but we also had many patients using discrete individualized doses, and always compounding capsules that did not contain lactose. Since then, the doses have become more varied, from the ultra-low dose (1-3 MICROgrams) and other patients with interstitial cystitis touching 12 mg, and some pain patients using multiple doses (four times daily) approaching a total dose of 15 mg! More importantly the individualized dosing has led us to improved patient benefit outcomes.

When we stay within the standardized old protocol we saw about 50% of patients having success, 20-25% saw some improvement with the final 25% seeing limited benefit, BUT when we optimize to individualized dosing and route (capsules, solutions, sublingual, topical), with the caveat of minimum three months of continued stable dosing, we saw much greater positive outcomes. This was not only reflected in symptoms of patients, but also in objective testing results.

Everything from ANAs, to TPO antibodies to WBCs and more. There is almost too much to describe in this short discussion, but it is the efforts of the LDN Research Trust (Linda Elsegood and her amazing team!!) and all of the health care practitioners and researchers that are moving the entire LDN movement forward, with profound changes in so many patients that it's overwhelming.

We all will continue to advocate for the safe utilization of LDN in the health care setting for our patients. Thank you for being such great advocates! Linda Elsegood - you are awesome!!

Ian S. Zagon, PhD, USA

I was stunned the day that my colleague came running up to me and said that "more is not better" - the higher doses of naltrexone were causing larger tumors and death, mice getting low doses of naltrexone were surviving. We had hypothesized the opposite - that more naltrexone would "cure" the tumored mice. This observation was serendipity.

Thus began decades of work establishing that the length of receptor blockade determined the response. We have shown that intermittent receptor blockade with low dose naltrexone results in lower cell proliferation and thus is beneficial for treatment of diseases with high levels of inflammatory cytokines (e.g., fibromyalgia, multiple sclerosis, and pain). Continuous receptor blockade with high doses of naltrexone results in accelerated proliferation.

After our initial discoveries in both cancer cells and developing rat brain were published in *Science* in 1983, clinicians capitalized on our discovery and termed the work "LDN" for treatment of patients. With the "cat out of the bag", a few small clinical trials were conducted but funding for a repurposed drug such as naltrexone was not easy to obtain.

Much of the translational work has occurred because of patients asking their physicians to try LDN. Today, LDN is widely used, but remains unauthorized by the FDA. My advice, remember that "more is not better."

Rehana Sajjad, MD, FACOG, USA

Many years ago, I read a book about low dose naltrexone and its effects on many autoimmune disorders. Since then I've taken LDN myself and prescribed it for my patients. I prescribe LDN for autoimmune diseases as well as for cancer, skin disorders such as psoriasis and neuropsychiatric disorders too.

I usually start my patients on 1.5 mg of LDN and then instruct them to increase to 4.5 mg. Some patients find better results at higher doses still. It's a very individual thing.

A few patients report sleep issues when starting LDN. These patients are instructed to take LDN in a morning or afternoon and this generally resolves these issues.

Patients reporting benefits from taking LDN are around 90%; very few have no benefit at all. LDN is a highly effective drug.

I see very good results on testing of patients on LDN. Auto antibodies often disappear. One patient with Graves' disease had very high antibodies and over time there were no TSI seen on testing. This patient has been on LDN four to five years now and is still doing well.

Scott Zashin, MD, USA

As a rheumatologist, I treat many conditions that affect patients' quality of life. Many deal with debilitating fatigue, pain or cognitive issues. While it is my job to diagnose and treat their problem, patients often will tell me about therapies that have helped them. Often, they described a treatment that I had not known. This was the case with low dose naltrexone.

A patient told me about it and wanted to try it. Unfortunately, this patient had a side effect from LDN which led to discontinuation. Nevertheless, I continued to hear about LDN from other patients and my own readings. I am happy to say I have prescribed the medication extensively over the past five years.

I became a doctor due to the personal satisfaction I received by being part of the health care team. Over the years I have seen dramatic improvements in patients who came to me after visiting many doctors who were unable to help them. I am always moved when they return for their follow-up visit expressing gratefulness to be feeling better, to have their life back due to LDN.

While most of my patients who take LDN have fibromyalgia, I noticed significant clinical benefit in my patients with Sjögren's syndrome and published a couple articles in a scientific journal detailing these cases. Sjögren's syndrome is a chronic autoimmune condition that is associated with dry eyes, dry mouth and often fatigue, joint/muscle pain and brain fog. Patients with Sjögren's are often prescribed a medication called hydroxychloroquine or Plaquenil. It is of interest that both medications share a similar mechanism of action involving the immune response.

Overall, it is heartening that so many of my patients have significant improvement in their quality of life while being treated with LDN.

Yusuf J.P. Saleeby, MD, USA

Low dose naltrexone (LDN) has been a part of my practice in functional medicine for over 15 years. Once relegated to those with autoimmune disease, vector borne illness such as Lyme disease, and cancer, it now has become a go-to for many disorders and as part of a prevention plan of action.

Since the COVID-19 pandemic and the data acquired by the researchers at the FLCCC it has become a mainstay of the chronic phases of COVID. PASC or long COVID, and now the injuries associated with the vaccinations, are now top priority disorders in which to start and keep patients on LDN until they recover.

The multiple mechanisms of action that LDN has an effect on the cell, mitochondria and organs is what is of benefit. I have personally used and still use LDN. I have been a student of this intervention to learn more for the benefit of the patients I take care of. While no one agent should be considered a panacea for everything nor a magic bullet, LDN comes very close to one. It is also one of the safest medications with a very low level of adverse side effects (ASE). As long as it is available it will make my very short list of good and safe pharmaceuticals.

I have been blessed to sit on the UK's LDN Research Trust medical advisory board for a number of years and be given the opportunity to research and lecture on LDN. I am honored to be one of the co-authors for the 3rd Volume of *The LDN Book*.

Natalie Walters, NP, AFMCP, CFMP, USA

I learned of LDN when my medical provider offered it to me in lieu of a biologic medication for ulcerative colitis in September 2022. I have had symptom relief and my calprotectin has also decreased from 2,022 to 300 since making numerous lifestyle changes and starting LDN. I continue on the LDN as it has unequivocally improved my symptoms and decreased inflammatory markers in my bloodwork.

I recently prescribed it for the first time for a 30-year-old male with neuropathic pain. After he took two doses of levofloxacin six years ago he has had chronic, unrelieved daily pain in his face, arms and legs which has been progressively worsening. He rates his pain level 10/10 prior to starting LDN and after just two weeks of LDN his pain level is 7-8/10.

This is an exciting tool that we have to help people with disease processes that usually have minimal treatment options.

Leonard Weinstock, MD, USA

I first heard about LDN in 2005. A pharmacist from a nearby compounding pharmacy stopped by my office and suggested I consider LDN for my patients with inflammation.

I started to prescribe LDN soon thereafter for patients with uncontrolled inflammatory bowel disease. Since 2005 LDN has been a major part of my medical practice and has been extended to patients with a host of inflammatory and painful conditions.

I generally start patients on 1 mg and increase every 4-7 days to get up to 4.5 mg. Then, for some, I add a 1 mg dose 12 hours later.

Only approximately 15% have side effects that prevent a full dose but some of these patients cannot tolerate the medicine at all. Around 50 – 60% of patients receive benefits from LDN.

In dermatologic disorders, the evidence of benefit is clear - their skin lesions get better (psoriasis and some dermatitis). In general care of multisystemic disease like mast cell activation syndrome, they just look and feel healthier.

My first patient was actually my wife. She had three years of suffering with restless legs syndrome. Night after night she had pain in her legs and a need to move. I treated her for small intestinal bacterial overgrowth and then followed it with LDN. For 12 years she has been in remission and also had relief from the frequent headaches she used to have.

A few words from my patients to describe their experience with LDN include:

"Amazing medicine - feel so much better."

"No migraines - first time in years."

"I forgot to refill it and after 2 days I felt all symptoms return which went away with resumption of the LDN."

I have extensive expertise with low dose naltrexone (LDN) in multiple inflammatory and autoimmune conditions. My research has been presented in national and international conferences and online interviews.

Emily Pratt, BSc, ND, USA

I have been prescribing low dose naltrexone (LDN) regularly for well over ten years now and I am still pleasantly surprised at its efficacy for chronic conditions, especially for those that have otherwise exhausted all other options to manage symptoms.

As a naturopathic physician my goal is to always seek out the underlying causation of disease, but coming from a research background (before becoming an ND), I always approach off-label uses and new treatments with a healthy level of skepticism. I still tell patients it is not a cure-all for their conditions, but I have seen patients have significant reduction in neurological, inflammatory, autoimmune, pain and/or mental/emotional symptoms. Some patients, specifically those with endometriosis, often experience a significant change within a few doses.

That being said, like any intervention, be it pharmaceutical or otherwise, it has to be the right patient, the right drug, the right dose and the right time. Thankfully in my practice, LDN has been a reliable intervention for the chronic symptoms of the "weird and wonderful" cases.

Angela Berry Koch, MS, Brazil

I first learned of LDN in 2012 from a naturopath in Seattle. It was then presented in an observational survey in 2015, by MyLymeData.org in the USA where more than 500 participants listed it above all other pain killers.

As a nutritionist in Brazil, I had collaborated with an MD who can write prescriptions, and used LDN for many patients. We always start out at low doses of 1-1.5 mg, depending on the patient history, and increase over many weeks. I have educated numerous practitioners in Brazil, coordinated with manipulation pharmacies on purity and neutrality of fillers, and promoted LDN benefits among an array of the health community.

We have seen noteworthy reduction in inflammatory markers such as CRP and ESR, and witnessed many patients, of many age groups, declare alleviation of inflammatory-related pain, heightened mood, and other positive results.

As a sufferer of idiopathic arthritis (probably related to COVID and my genetics, hereditary alpha tryptasemia), I have taken LDN for two years.

I have found it combines well with compounded ketotifen and the combination has both allowed for sustained alleviation of joint symptoms, as well as better sleep.

I feel fortunate to live in Brazil where the cost of compounding is minimal. The dosage of 6 mg a day is costing only about US$15 a month. This is very fortunate and makes LDN accessible to many. I believe other countries should follow suit.

Phil Boyle, MB, BCh, NUI, MICGP, MRCGP, CFCP, Ireland

I was already familiar with naltrexone, the opioid antagonist used to treat patients with drug addictions but I first heard about LDN from my sister, Mary Boyle Bradley. Her neurologist in New York, Dr. Bernard Bihari, prescribed LDN to treat her husband's MS. He responded so well to treatment; she wrote a book to share his story and promote this novel treatment.

I am a fertility doctor, but I started to prescribe LDN for some of my patients who had autoimmune illnesses and most responded favourably to treatment with reduced inflammation, increased energy, improved mood and lifting of "brain fog."

Gradually I began to recommend LDN for some of my infertility patients and I noticed additional benefits. With LDN they had less period pain and PMS, and menstrual cycles became more regular. LDN was especially helpful for endometriosis. Initially I discontinued LDN during pregnancy, but negative symptoms would return and miscarriage seemed to be more frequent, so I have given LDN during pregnancy since 2007.

Today, I estimate 50% of my patients use LDN to treat infertility and most continue it during pregnancy. Over 1,000 of my patients have used LDN in pregnancy and clinically both mother and baby do very well. We have a low incidence of prematurity, pre-eclampsia or low birth weight. I suspect LDN contributes significantly to our positive outcomes.

I usually consider LDN if a patient is clinically endorphin deficient. If she has two or more of the following: painful periods, brown menstrual bleeding, endometriosis, fatigue, low mood, anxiety or autoimmune illness, I suspect low endorphins and recommend LDN.

I usually start with 3 mg nightly for the first week and try 4.5 mg thereafter. I adjust the dose as needed and discontinue it if vivid dreams or sleep disturbance persist beyond the first 7-10 days. This means endorphins are too high and we either lower the dose or stop it altogether. I don't use more than 4.5 mg, but can go as low as 2 mg strength.

Clinically seven out of every ten patients seem to respond favourably to LDN treatment - this is much higher than expected for placebo which will see improvement 30% of the time. I judge effectiveness based on what patients tell me, rather than any specific blood test or scan. I previously had two patients with progressive MS who had no progression on MRI after five years of treatment, but I rarely see MS patients.

My typical patient presents with low mood, fatigue, PMS and period pain. In addition to LDN, I recommend dietary changes - low carbs with minimal dairy and wheat. It is best to avoid vegetable oils and switch to coconut oil for cooking. I also recommend vitamin D3 4000 IU daily with a good Omega-3 supplement (EPA 700 mg+) to reduce inflammation. I usually see them back after eight weeks of treatment and repeatedly find a dramatic improvement in most of these negative symptoms.

It is common, and good practice, to use off-label medications. Remember to absolutely avoid morphine when using naltrexone as it interacts badly. Also, better to avoid codeine and take minimal alcohol while on LDN treatment.

Steve Hoffart, PharmD, USA

I heard about LDN at a PCCA event. We compounded a small amount of LDN from 2010 to 2017. In 2017, we hosted a prescriber education event taught by Sebastian Denison (PCCA) and our LDN compounding exploded. In 2018, I attended the LDN Research Trust annual conference and greatly expanded my knowledge on LDN to better help prescribers and patients on how to use LDN in their practice and their health journey.

We start most patients on 0.5 mg to 1.5 mg of LDN and titrate up slowly from there. Lately, as we care for patients that are medically fragile, we are starting at lower doses in the 0.25 mg to 0.5 mg range to allow for slow titration and minimize side effects.

The highest daily dose of LDN we dispense is 12-15 mg. We typically see the higher doses split as multiple times a day.

We greatly reduce the incidence of side effects by starting low and going slow. The side effect incidence runs approximately 10% or less for our patients. Side effects are mild but the most common is sleep disturbances that can be corrected by dosing earlier in the day. The second most common side effect is GI issues related to constipation. To prevent this problem, we can compound LDN in a sublingual or transdermal dosage form.

Better than 80% of the patients we start on LDN see some benefit from the medication.

Items to monitor to measure a patient's success on LDN include a complete thyroid panel including antibodies, hs-CRP, IL-6, and other markers of inflammation or other autoimmune conditions.

One of our first patients on LDN was suffering with Crohn's disease and was on a biologic to control symptoms. The practitioner started the patient on LDN and implemented lifestyle and dietary changes. When we completed a follow-up visit with the patient at ten months, the patient's Crohn's disease had improved to a point that the prescriber had removed the biologic, and the patient was only using LDN to control their Crohn's disease. This is quite remarkable when considering the healthcare dollar savings and the reduced side effect profile by eliminating the biologic.

Since adding compounded low dose naltrexone to our practice in 2017, it has been the single most impactful medication in assisting our patients with numerous complex medical conditions. As we get a better understanding of how most of our known disease processes are driven by inflammation, LDN becomes the natural fit to assist and reduce inflammation and thus be an integral part of improving the health and wellness of our patients.

Being a pharmacist and developing close relationships with patients during their wellness journeys, LDN is commonly mentioned as the biggest addition to therapy that improved their quality of life.

With great outcomes, minimal side effects, and low costs, LDN provides a tremendous and unique therapeutic option to help patients to achieve positive outcomes. The LDN Research Trust has been integral in compiling, educating, and sharing information on the vast number of conditions benefited by LDN. The future looks bright for the growth of LDN use in more and more medical conditions.

Debora Chelson, NMD, USA

I have been using LDN in my practice for around 13 years, with more success than failures.

There is a family history of dementia in my family, so I have been using LDN for about two years now, to decrease inflammation, and to keep it from getting to my brain. My head is less foggy, and the health of my feet has improved. I had lost the nail on my big toes many times over the years from backpacking. Once they grew back, they were fine, until the warmer months. As soon as I started wearing sandals and went barefoot, I would get toenail fungus and would battle it all the way until it got cold again, I tried everything, and nothing worked. This spring and summer there have been no issues, only normal toenails. That is important to me, and the only thing I can attribute this to is the LDN.

I have a patient who is a 45-year-old female who had been dealing with Crohn's, gastroparesis, reactive arthritis, and chronic diarrhea. When she was in her twenties she worked as a vet tech and spent her days applying flea and tick solution on dogs, with no gloves. She suffered from painful joints and migraines most of the time. There were only a handful of foods she could eat that did not exacerbate her symptoms. Between the pain, diarrhea, and fatigue she was limited in her daily activities.

I was not certain the LDN would be of any benefit due to her compromised GI tract. She was able to titrate to 3 mg with minimal issues, and we agreed to meet in three months to assess her health status. She reported that her gastroparesis was being held at bay with the LDN, and most of her pain was gone. The diarrhea had decreased, and she was able to add many more foods into her diet with no issues. She stated this was the best she has felt in about ten years. She has started running a few days a week and was able to spend four days at Disneyworld without any health issues.

I had an otherwise healthy and active 80-year-old female patient come to me with osteoarthritis in both hands, causing so much pain and stiffness, it was almost impossible for her to do anything with her hands. They were so swollen that she had to remove her wedding ring.

Because she had waited so long to do anything about her condition, I really had to hold her hand through the first six weeks, until she felt the pain subsiding a bit. Currently she is still on 4 mg of LDN, and she has no more pain in her hands. Best of all she can wear her wedding ring again.

Kristen Cardamone, DO, USA

I first began using LDN in about 2017 after researching more about it at the suggestion of my friend and colleague, compound pharmacist, Dr. John Kim.

In my earlier prescribing days, I would generally start patients at about 4.5 mg and the majority would tolerate the dose well and have quite dramatic results. However, I noticed that some of my more sensitive, autoimmune patients could not tolerate that dose. Once I started at 0.5 mg and titrated weekly to about 4.5 mg, altering formulations between troche and liquid as needed, this chronic, often complex, patient population had dramatic results.

Overall, I would estimate that about 90% of my patients note dramatic improvement, and the small percentage that do not is largely due to premature discontinuation of LDN due to impatience, an underlying structural pain generator, such as severe spinal stenosis, or a GI intolerance issue.

Over the years, I also started noticing not only ESR and CRP levels dropping in many autoimmune patients, but also diabetics having normalization of their glucose and HbA1c in some cases.

I have so many examples of patients with amazing results from LDN. One more recent case involves a colleague who suffered from post-COVID full body urticaria and facial edema. She saw an ED doc, PMD, ENT and an allergist without definitive diagnosis or effective treatment. I started her on 0.5 mg LDN and titrated 0.5 mg each week to 4.5 mg nightly and her symptoms resolved by about six weeks.

I also have countless other patients, many female, who were dismissed as having fibromyalgia or being told there was "nothing else to offer" who have also since reported "life changing" results with LDN.

LDN has truly been a game changer for my practice and I urge all those physicians who are unfamiliar with this safe, simple treatment to become knowledgeable in prescribing it. You will not be disappointed in your patient outcomes, and your patients will be extremely grateful.

Personally, I have suffered from chronic fatigue since my early 30s, likely as a result of the perfect storm of stress, Epstein-Barr, Lyme disease, followed by mycoplasma pneumonia and finally, more recently having COVID twice. It was even more frustrating since I had the knowledge and medical resources to trial almost every imaginable alternative and traditional treatment, yet I still could not find a great solution for my fatigue until I incorporated low dose naltrexone. I've been taking LDN 4.5 mg since about 2020 with excellent results, including during the COVID pandemic. I have not experienced the often severe bouts of fatigue that I used to suffer prior to starting LDN. I noticed results almost immediately upon starting, but definitely within the first month. LDN has also been a life saver for me as a busy medical professional and mom.

Tania Tyles Dempsey, MD, ABIHM, USA

In 2011, after I started my own integrative and personalized medical practice, I had a patient who brought LDN to my attention because she wanted my opinion on whether it would be helpful to treat her Hashimoto's thyroiditis. I had heard of the drug before but didn't have experience at the time. I did a lot of research and decided that I felt comfortable prescribing it for the patient. I started her on 1.5 mg of LDN, which is what I understood at the time was the proper starting dosage. I slowly titrated her to 3 mg and then 4.5 mg and over the next year her thyroid antibodies decreased and her thyroid function improved.

While this is only a n=1, I saw the potential for the drug and with additional research began trialing it in other appropriate patients with thyroid conditions at first, and then in other conditions. As my understanding of a complex, multisystem illness known as MCAS deepened, it became even clearer to me that LDN could be an important tool in the treatment of MCAS. What I have seen is that a large percentage, I would estimate about 75-80% of patients do quite well with LDN; some find LDN to be the game changer in controlling their MCAS symptoms, while others find LDN a great adjunct to a comprehensive MCAS-targeted protocol. However, about 15-20% of my patients do not seem to tolerate LDN. While it is not clear yet how to identify which patients are those who will have a negative response to the drug, it does seem that these patients are primarily having reactions that are driven by their dysfunctional mast cells.

Regarding dosing, I usually start at lower dosages than I did when I first started prescribing the drug 12 years ago. I commonly have my patients start at 0.5 mg, but I have also used much lower dosages, like 0.1 mg, in my very sensitive patients. I have found that many of my patients seem to tolerate it better when taken in the morning as opposed to the evening, but I have a select few who do better taking it in the evening. I also typically titrate up slowly. The majority of patients wind up around 4.5-5 mg but the maximum dosage I have used to date is 9 mg.

For the patient population that I treat, I don't always see specific markers change on lab work but I have certainly seen decreasing autoantibody titers or decreased inflammatory markers in some patients. The improvement that I see in patients who have a positive response to LDN is in their tolerance to the environment, with less activation of their mast cells.

Overall, LDN is a great tool in the armamentarium for treating immune dysregulation, including conditions such as MCAS.

Apple Bodemer, MD, USA

I have been prescribing LDN for seven or eight years. I personally have been taking it for about four years (off and on if I am honest).

I learned about LDN from a patient who I was seeing for skin cancer screening. She was in later mid-life and one day when she came in, she told me all about how much she hikes and kayaks. I glanced at her "problem list" in the electronic medical record and saw multiple sclerosis. I was a bit surprised because she was so active and I asked her how long she had been living with that diagnosis. I was shocked to hear that she had been diagnosed 25 years earlier!

I have taken care of many people who have MS and I have never seen anyone able to maintain that level of activity. It was almost unbelievable to me, so I asked her what she was doing that might be different from most people with MS. She told me that a few years into her diagnosis, she found a practitioner who prescribed LDN. She felt that was making the difference!

I was so curious that I could barely get to the end of my clinic that day. I was really excited to learn more about LDN. That was the beginning of my journey as an LDN prescriber. I have seen it help so many conditions! Some that I intended to treat (like psoriasis, eczema, lichen planopilaris, vitiligo, alopecia areata), and others that have ended up being pleasant side effects (such as decreased cravings for carbs and alcohol, better mood, improved sleep, less anxiety).

My personal experience came a bit later. I have struggled with some joint discomfort that shows up when I am stressed and not taking good care of myself. It never has fallen into any specific diagnostic category, but I suspect I have a tendency for something autoimmune related. I would go see my acupuncturist for 4-6 treatments when it was flared up, which was usually once or twice a year.

After a few years of prescribing LDN and seeing really great results, I decided to give it a try myself. For three years I took it regularly and didn't have a single flare. Life got busy and I got lax about taking it. I ended up going off it for about a year – for no particular reason except for I kept forgetting to get it refilled or forgot to take it. The joint discomfort started to come back, and I have been back on it for about three months. My joint discomfort is better and improving.

My intention is to be on LDN long term – I have seen the impact it has on my symptoms and that those symptoms came back when I stopped. It is such a safe therapy and having seen people who have been on it for over 30 years at this point, makes me feel even more confident that this is something that can be a long-term therapeutic option.

Carol Knowles, PA-C, USA

I have had several successes using LDN in my pain management practice in a conventional orthopedic practice. It has helped patients with musculoskeletal pain such as arthritis and sciatica. Where I have been very pleased with results have been in the more complicated patients with autoimmune arthritis, GI issues such as gastroparesis and of course with fibromyalgia. I was limited with using LDN due to the percentage of my patient population already on opioids for their chronic pain.

I have recently left the orthopedic practice and have been the pain management provider at a Veteran's Health Administration facility. The VA system has been implementing a new pain management initiative. One of the goals of this VA initiative is to decrease the amount of opioids prescribed for chronic pain. Naturally, I thought that LDN would be a great tool for use in managing chronic and complicated pain issues with our veterans. I have been very excited to learn that there are other providers within the VA system who are aware of LDN and are also interested in prescribing it to their patients. While the VA system does not have LDN on their formulary, there are some VA pharmacies around the country that have been able to order it from compounding pharmacies. I am currently working on getting my VA to have LDN available for my patients.

For every conversation that I have about LDN with a patient, I pull up the LDN Research Trust website on my computer and show patients how they can do their own further reading on the medication. The extensive "List of conditions treated" on the website is always a great teaching tool. I currently have a female veteran on LDN for her chronic, widespread pain and fatigue that has been labelled fibromyalgia. She has lost weight and has been able to exercise with reduced pain since starting the LDN. She was willing for me to give her a hard copy prescription that she takes to a compounding pharmacy outside of the VA.

I feel like employing LDN in a widespread way within the VA system could be a game changer for treating complicated patients with chronic pain and multiple comorbidities such as autoimmune issues, substance use disorder etc. I also feel that LDN use within the VA healthcare system will be a tremendous opportunity for more patients, practitioners and health care policy makers to be aware of the benefits of this medication. I hope to document my results with patients and collaborate with my peers around the country who are also using LDN with their patients.

I have appreciated the LDN Research Trust for its very helpful information on LDN and I look forward to becoming the "LDN expert" within the VA.

Jerry Meloche, PharmD, USA

My wife Lisa and I have owned a compounding pharmacy since 2005, and because we have always had the opportunity to work with functional/holistic prescribers for all of that time, we have been compounding LDN for most of that time - so almost 18 years.

After hearing of the many successful experiences of our patients over the years, my wife and I pushed our physician to prescribe it for us - not for anything in particular, but for all of the general health benefits it had to offer.

One of our most memorable patients was the husband of a veterinary technician at a local specialty veterinary clinic. She explained to me that he had been diagnosed with Crohn's disease and that his physician was "strongly" suggesting the use of biologics to "treat" his condition. She also explained that he was very hesitant to start that therapy due to the possibly serious adverse effects associated with its use.

I generally explained LDN to her, gave her the LDN Research Trust website address, and told her that if her husband wanted more information about LDN to call me. Surprisingly, he called the next day and we had a long conversation about LDN's possible benefits, and maybe more importantly, its lack of serious adverse side effects. He subsequently contacted his physician (who, turns out, was a local "more open minded" physician that we were very familiar with) who called in his first prescription for LDN.

He picked it up the next day, and was very excited to start his adventure and healing process. After about three months, he came in to pick up his refill and informed me that many of his more troublesome symptoms were subsiding and he was feeling better. A few months later, he reported that most of his symptoms had gone away and that his physician was very happy with his progress and was happy to continue his LDN therapy.

Along with the above patient, we have had dozens of success stories with LDN. Many patients have reported reduction of symptoms from a multitude of conditions, including Hashimoto's thyroiditis, GI inflammatory conditions, autoimmune skin conditions, various pain syndromes with multiple causes (osteo- and rheumatoid arthritis, CRPS, neuropathies, etc.), and weight loss, to name just a few.

As local independent pharmacy owners, pharmacists, and human beings, we will continue to advocate for, recommend, compound, and personally take LDN, due to the huge benefits and general lack of harm that LDN offers. As I tell every prospective and interested patient and physician, "LDN should be in the water we drink."

Thank you to the LDN Research Trust for raising awareness about LDN.

Debora Donahue, APRN-BC, USA

I first heard about LDN through my MS patients who were under the care of a specialist in Orlando. They discussed how LDN was keeping their symptoms under control and had prevented flares for years. They were so happy to not be taking strong drugs. LDN had given them their life back.

I started prescribing LDN about three years ago on a select few patients with Hashimoto's thyroiditis and high antibody levels. I did see improvement in the numbers, but they did not seem to really feel any physical manifestations of taking the LDN.

I then decided to try using LDN on patients with newly-diagnosed positive ANA tests and symptoms of pain. They often did not want the rheumatologists' drugs, and would instead request to trial LDN; it worked great.

My normal dosing is 4-4.5 mg nightly. I have a few patients who requested to go higher, so they are on 5-6 mg nightly and seeing great results. They were seeing OK results at 4 mg. These patients also tend to be higher BMI.

I believe 90-95% of my patients see benefits with LDN. Only a few have said they never saw results. The others who may have stopped did so because of sleep issues, even though it was working.

I do see an improvement in the thyroid antibody levels along with CRP.

I have patients using LDN for GI issues – in particular, one for UC and another for collagenous colitis. Both of these people had been experiencing diarrhea, urgency and even occasional leakage which was terribly embarrassing. Not to mention the "gurgles" in the intestines during an office meeting or with friends. Both are on LDN, seeing dramatic improvements in bowel frequency, consistency, cramping/ bloating and gas.

I have another patient who has had severe psoriasis for many years. Her entire back was quite thickened skin, very rough, irritated and uncomfortable. None of her specialists had been able to make a significant improvement. The LDN was able to stop the progression, stop the inflammation and discomfort, and enable her to return to work duties feeling much improved.

Other providers and specialists need to receive information about how LDN works, how safe it is, and how effective it is for so many people. I provide my patients a handout to give to their other providers so there is no confusion as to why they are taking naltrexone.

Debbie Judd, ARNP, USA

LDN is an amazing, miraculous medication. I prescribe it more than any other medication in my practice and most of my patients are taking it, with great success.

I am a nurse practitioner who owns and operates a functional medicine clinic in Spokane, WA. Our providers have been prescribing LDN for over 18 years. We treat the full spectrum of chronic disease processes. Autoimmune diseases, cancers, MS, Parkinsons, mold toxicity, GI issues, chronic pain and inflammation, chronic fatigue, MCAS and Lyme disease are some of the conditions we treat with LDN. This medication has helped improve the quality of life for our patients.

From the young to the elderly, across the lifespan, LDN helps give patients back their birthright: to be as healthy as possible given the health circumstances they are experiencing.

Dawn Ipsen, PharmD, USA

As a compounding pharmacist in Washington state, I've had the privilege to help patients with customized doses of low dose naltrexone (LDN) for nearly 20 years. In that time, I helped solidify dosing protocols and best practices to achieve optimal patient outcomes. In addition, I became a national educator and speaker for patients and prescribers seeking to utilize such an innovative and effective therapeutic tool.

Initially, pharmacists such as myself specifically thought of LDN when treating conditions such as multiple sclerosis, fibromyalgia, and Crohn's disease. However, as our learning and experience evolved, we realized there was much more to LDN as a therapy. Now that we have a better understanding of the functions and potential mechanisms of action, I see LDN as a helpful therapy for many chronic conditions that are inflammation based. This most recently includes autoimmune conditions, thyroid disorders, post-COVID syndrome, traumatic brain injury, irritable bowel disease and many, many others.

Our patient, CH shared with us her experience with taking LDN for long COVID. She states that, "I started with one pill for a week, and then I slowly moved up. Once I was at that higher amount the changes I noticed were that my heart rate totally normalized. I don't have exhaustion anymore and I have more energy than before I had kids. Huge change there! My body aches also went away. I had severe adrenal fatigue onset right before COVID started, which made body aches worse. The LDN has helped all these symptoms resolve. The energy change was huge, and the gallbladder pain completely resolved almost immediately after getting up to that full dose."

Primarily, best practices include thorough assessment of the patient's condition for causes and specifically cellular dysfunctions. Then an assessment of LDN risk versus benefit is helpful when initiating LDN therapy. Generally, LDN appears to be of low risk with potentially high benefit for many patients. Furthermore, it is critical to work with a medical team that includes practitioners familiar with and experts in prescribing LDN, as well as a compounding pharmacy with expertise in quality, accuracy, and patient individuality. Customization of the dose, dosage form, and time of dosing is critical for successful treatment.

Our pharmacists are experts in helping patients who require therapies for chronic illnesses. We strive to help patients live their best lives through innovative and personalized medications. We make the medicine fit the patients' needs!

Amy Smith-Bassett, APRN, USA

My APRN provider recommended LDN to me about eight years ago for Hashimoto's thyroiditis and chronic inflammation. It made a big difference in my lab results and how I felt physically. I no longer have positive thyroid antibodies!

I began prescribing LDN around 2018 and have continued to do so since then. Many of my patients have experienced benefits and healing from taking LDN. My views on dosage are changing; previously I would start with 1.5 mg and taper up to 4.5 mg. Since becoming a LDN Specialist and reading/listening to new information, I am beginning to prescribe 0.5 mg and having patients taper up slowly to find their "happy place." The highest dose I have yet prescribed is 4.5 mg, although I am now willing to consider higher doses. Anecdotally, I would say two thirds of patients have benefits and I am wondering if the remaining patients would improve with smaller dose adjustments and closer follow-up.

Often inflammatory markers show improvement, sometimes even before the patient notices a response. I've seen ANA results improve, thyroid antibodies improve, sed rate and CRP improve, and more.

I take LDN for Hashimoto's hypothyroidism and general inflammation. My symptoms have been subtle and ongoing for years. I wouldn't say my life was severely affected by my symptoms but I didn't feel well. My integrative APRN offered LDN and at first I was skeptical. I had already been taking compounded thyroid medication and had cut out inflammatory foods. I believe at the time of starting LDN I was only taking thyroid medication. It was not difficult to obtain a prescription since we have a fantastic compounding pharmacy nearby.

I started taking LDN in 2016 and believe that I tapered up from 1.5 mg to 3 mg to 4.5 mg. I currently take 4.5 mg. I do not experience any side effects. At first I may have had an increase in vivid dreams, but this is not atypical for me anyway. LDN definitely relieved some of my inflammatory symptoms (rosacea, joint pain, fatigue) and has continued to help with inflammation in my lab markers. At one time I did have a positive ANA, this is now negative. Currently I take thyroid medication, bio-identical hormones, and LDN. I am so grateful my provider suggested this amazing tool so many years ago.

Ginny Isbell, PharmD, USA

I've worked with LDN since 2006 and have seen multiple patients with many different disease states use it with success. We often see LDN prescribed for Hashimoto's and have become accustomed to patients coming back to tell us they feel better or their lab results have improved.

I remember one particular patient (diagnosed with Hashimoto's) coming into our pharmacy to get her low dose naltrexone. Since this was her first time getting LDN from our pharmacy I counselled her on the medication. She had been taking LDN for a while, but didn't really know if it was helping when she decided to start getting it from our pharmacy. We discussed how to take it and the minor side effects that might be seen. She explained she had never experienced any of the sleep disturbances that she had been told might occur with low dose naltrexone. She also explained that she was not sure if LDN was working for her because her thyroid antibodies remained elevated and she had not really noticed any changes while taking it.

I explained that we usually had great success with LDN bringing thyroid antibodies down and asked if she had also removed gluten from her diet. She was very knowledgeable about autoimmune conditions and was sticking to a very strict diet. We talked further and then she left with her medication. A few days after she started taking LDN from our pharmacy she called stating she did experience the wakening for the first time when she started taking LDN from our pharmacy and was hopeful that it was working. I explained how fillers and the quality of the active ingredient can make a huge difference in the absorption and effects of a compounded prescription.

A few weeks later she called again and let me know that her thyroid antibodies had come down for the first time. She was very excited because she had been eating clean for a long time and finally, by switching to our pharmacy, her antibodies had normalized.

I believe that we all have the ability to heal and hope that others who are experiencing chronic health problems will continue looking for answers until they find them. As a compounding pharmacist for over 17 years, I have seen over and over how quality products (nutrients, food and compounded prescriptions) can make a huge difference in our health.

We must choose to make our decisions based on quality, not cost, if we expect these therapies to work.

Following the work that the LDN Research Trust does, and going through the LDN Specialist course twice has taught me that one dose/ one protocol of LDN does not work for everyone. Many times, we have to work with patients to adjust their dose or dosage form to get the best results for an individual.

If you have a condition that has not been helped with traditional medications, I encourage you to reach out to someone who is knowledgeable about LDN and who will listen to you and treat you like the individual you are. I believe there is help out there for you. Be well.

Brooke Hogg, PharmD, USA

I discovered LDN back in 2008 when I had the opportunity to do a compounding rotation with a pharmacy. When I started, Skip Lenz was in the middle of doing an LDN survey for a UCLA multiple sclerosis conference he was presenting at. It was a post-surveillance survey for patients that had been on LDN for six months or longer. I contacted approximately 200 patients to ask them a series of questions pertaining to their therapeutic outcome while taking LDN.

After speaking with these patients, it opened my eyes to a whole new realm of treatment other than what we learn in school. To hear patients talk about being able to garden again or ice skate was the most liberating experience. You don't learn about this therapy in school. Compounding opened doors for me clinically that I never would have learned in retail or hospital. Moving forward 15 years later, I never left this pharmacy. I have been the managing pharmacist pretty much my whole career.

For a long time we have used the standard titration starting with 1.5 mg, to 3 mg, and a maintenance dose of 4.5 mg. The last five to eight years we are seeing more and more chemical sensitivity. We are able to accommodate these patients with a lower milligram. We also have patients with autism, or CRPS, that may benefit more from dosing at 6 mg to 9 mg or the dose split up taken twice daily.

In my experience, when LDN is taken at bedtime, 98% of our patients, who have been on LDN for six months or more, barely get sick and if they do, the colds are cut in half. This is a really important characteristic LDN has when using this in patients with autoimmune issues, cancer, or HIV.

Diagnostics are really helpful for clinicians and patients. Labs show decreases in antibody levels and sedimentation rates or other inflammatory markers. We see decreased plaque formation in the brain with MRI. When the rectum is scoped the health of the tissue imaging is improved. The list goes on.

In a nutshell, having thousands of patients on LDN speaks for itself. Being a part of our patients' journey and improving their quality of life is the most rewarding gift. I love what I do. It is a constant learning process.

Linda Bluestein, MD, USA

I first heard about LDN from a pain management physician colleague who felt I might benefit from taking it. That was around 2016, after seven years of chronic pain that greatly impacted my quality of life and ability to function as a physician anesthesiologist. I believe that LDN is the single most important medication that gave me my life (and career) back.

I never thought my health would be better in my late 50s than it was in my mid-40s.

I started prescribing LDN in 2017 when I opened my integrative pain management practice, which focuses on those with symptomatic joint hypermobility and connective tissue disorders like the Ehlers-Danlos syndromes. I usually prescribe 1.5 mg and titrate from there up to 4.5-6 mg every evening. I start significantly lower in selected patients and some patients benefit from twice daily dosing. I have seen patients as high as 7 mg twice daily although I have never prescribed dosing that high.

About 80% of my patients experience some degree of improvement. The results are often dramatic with patients reporting that they have more energy, better focus, less headaches, less widespread body pain, and improved quality of life.

I have hypermobile Ehlers-Danlos syndrome, Tarlov cyst, and have had multiple orthopedic injuries and surgeries. I have had symptoms throughout my entire life. Before I started LDN and the other components of my comprehensive treatment plan (movement, nutrition, education, sleep, addressing psychosocial aspects, and supplements), the quality of my life was very poor. I was experiencing daily severe pain, fatigue, poor sleep, decreased appetite, and suboptimal mood.

After starting LDN, my symptoms gradually improved. Over time, I continue to be able to increase my activity level. In 2010, I spent an entire month on the couch and the other day I completed an eight mile hike with significant elevation gain. I was offered a spinal cord stimulator and am so grateful I declined that invasive procedure.

I currently take LDN 6 mg every evening and have not experienced any adverse effects. I have vivid dreams but I find them enjoyable. I am incredibly grateful to be able to function and live a good quality of life. I still have physical limitations but I can do fun activities and feel good most all of the time.

Cory Tichauer, ND, USA

Since discovering the benefits of low dose naltrexone over 15 years ago, it has firmly established itself as a foundational treatment in my medical practice. LDN's ability to calm the expression of proinflammatory cytokines and alleviate a cycle of immune inflammation makes it almost ubiquitously applicable in the treatment of complex chronic illness. Whether treating for an underlying infectious illness, disturbed immune dysfunction or a progressive inflammatory disorder, I have found that LDN provides a stout base for shifting the patient response toward resolution and recovery.

Graduating in 1996 with a BA in Neurobiology from Cornell University, I had always intended to become a physician. My interest was rooted in helping to solve the puzzle of chronic illness that, like cancer, was growing in both scope and complexity by the year. This focus led me away from an allopathic education and instead saw me enroll in a naturopathic medical school where I would be better equipped with a vitalistic, rather than mechanistic, understanding of human physiology and treatment. Reflecting 20 years later, this proved to be a pivotal decision, as I have successfully treated this underserved population of patients.

Currently, I treat a wide range of conditions that fall into this category including tick-borne illness, autoimmune conditions, mast cell activation syndrome, neurodegenerative diagnoses and environmental illness. The ability of low dose naltrexone to shift the immune system away from fulminating (adaptive) immune inflammation toward an effective cell-mediated immunity has shown to be the unifying central principle in all of these wide-ranging situations. Whether the goal is to clear an intracellular infection or to reduce immune activation, the capacity of LDN to balance TH1/TH2 T-cell reactivity, ameliorate neuroinflammation and improve immune tolerance via T-reg and IL-10 stimulation, has made it an indispensable tool in my practice.

John Chinwe, MD, USA

I first heard about low dose naltrexone approximately five years ago, from a patient of mine. I am always open to learning about safe therapies for my patients, and so I embarked on my own research, reading up as much as I could about LDN, Dr. Bihari, and the compounding pharmacies available to me. The LDN Research Trust was one of the resources I utilized at the time.

I tried LDN first on a patient with autoimmune disease and chronic pain. I was pleased with the positive feedback reported by the patient, and have had good results with the drug ever since.

Typically, I start my patients on a dose between 0.25-0.75 mg depending on the patient's history. The highest dose of LDN I use is 4.5 mg. I would say no less than 97% of my patients see benefits from LDN.

Most of the improvement I follow is based on a combination of the patient's self-reported decrease or elimination of symptoms, improvement on physical examination, and decrease in markers depending on the condition, for example, normalized TSH levels in a case of Hashimoto's thyroiditis, and decreased ESR levels.

An example of a recent case is: A woman in her thirties with rheumatoid arthritis and hypothyroidism, who contacted my practice at the start of the year. She had previously been on LDN in another state, but had been off it for some time since her move. Her symptoms were moderate-severe pain in the hands, hips and knees, which interfered with her daily activities. She was placed on LDN following my individualized prescribed titration, and by six months follow up, has resolution of her joint pains. She uses thyroid hormone replacement and had some issues with dose adjustment which her endocrinologist assists her with. On her last follow up, her thyroid markers were better controlled. She reported no side effects from LDN.

A small number of patients cannot tolerate LDN, however with close monitoring, I have found it to be a safe and effective therapy in combination with other appropriate therapies, in the treatment of musculoskeletal manifestations of autoimmune diseases, post-COVID symptoms aka long COVID, fibromyalgia and other chronic pain syndromes.

Vince Meo, RPh, USA

I first heard about LDN when I started working at the pharmacy three years ago. Practicing pharmacy as a retail pharmacist my whole career, I immediately was intrigued and initially thought patients must be getting some kind of placebo effect; then I soon realized that I had a lot more to learn than I thought.

One day, I was talking to a patient who was taking high doses of opioids for years for chronic pain. Over time, working with her physician, she was able to wean off her opioids while titrating her dose of LDN. Now her pain is tolerable with LDN alone.

It is very interesting to see the variations of knowledge amongst the providers and patients regarding LDN. It is humbling to be able to provide knowledge, especially given the new approach toward LDN discussed by many providers at the LDN conference. Not basing dose on a standard for every patient but realizing that all patients are different regarding sensitivity to drugs, as well as metabolism and receptor differences.

Some of our patients have done their research and know exactly what they want. For instance, why they feel they do not want a tablet vs a capsule, need for a specific filler and exactly why they need LDN. On the other hand, many of our patients have many questions about their new LDN script.

Many patients are excited, some are frustrated because they have already exhausted many of the conventional treatments. We sometimes get patients starting LDN again after a failed attempt usually due to side effects, which is a problem that can be solved by correct dosing/titrating or even the time of day that LDN is taken.

Regardless, it is a pleasure to be able to supply them with information on why the medication needs to be compounded, how the medication works, side effects, the difference between the different dosage forms available and why they would choose one over another depending on allergies/sensitivities, disease states i.e., absorption issues/GI sensitivities/mast cell. As well as any other information they may need to help them be successful with their LDN therapy.

Michelle Moser, RPh, FAPC, FACA, FACVP, USA

I first heard about LDN during a pain conference in the early 2000s. I had known about naltrexone as the medication that we use for addiction but was intrigued by the properties of low doses.

As I read more and more about LDN, spoke with other compounding pharmacies across the US and Canada, I began compounding and hearing patients review LDN as "changing their lives," and allowing them to "feel normal" again.

It became very apparent that the dosing regimens needed to be tailored to the needs of the individual. As the practice of pharmacy has evolved, we see more attention being paid to genetics, autoimmune root causes, how to improve chronic disease outcomes and keep people healthy for as long as possible.

Over the years, we have seen an improvement from 50% of patients having benefited from LDN to over 85% now seeing improvement! Some patients are on 0.1 mg once or twice a day or up to 6 mg! Most people report that their symptoms improve over time, they may be able to reduce the number of medications that they are taking, or that they can now return to activities that they had been forced to abandon.

It's hard to pinpoint which patient will benefit from LDN, as their backgrounds, their medical conditions and length of chronic issues all vary so widely. In my pharmacy, we see people who have medical issues that are not being resolved with traditional medications, who have spent years, if not decades, searching for help, and who are willing to try this low dose, low side effect, low risk, low cost medication to "see" how it will work out. Most are pleasantly surprised to find benefit over a relatively short period of time. Their prescribers are often surprised too!

Working directly with patients and providers to find the individual "happy" dose is how patients' successful outcomes are found. This takes commitment and communication from a knowledgeable medical professional to ensure healthy outcomes.

Being an LDN Specialist has allowed me to continue my education on the latest information available on LDN through the LDN Research Trust.

Mona Morstein, ND, DHANP, VNMI, USA

I'm Dr. Mona Morstein, a naturopathic physician of 35 years, in Mesa, AZ. I learned about LDN at conferences on SIBO (small intestine bacterial overgrowth). LDN was discussed both in terms of being a mild prokinetic, which can prevent SIBO from returning once it's been eradicated, and as a help for those who have vinculin antibodies. Vinculin antibodies can be a common cause of SIBO as they prevent the small intestine from moving forward appropriately.

LDN was discussed as helping reduce autoimmune reactions in the body. I started using LDN then, after time learning it's a bit better to titrate up dosage than start with higher doses at first. I always dose 1.5 mg, and recommend one capsule at bedtime for a week, then 2 capsules at bedtime for a week, then three capsules at bedtime for a week. Patients then let me know which dose worked best for them and I then prescribe that dose for a year.

I now use LDN for many autoimmune medical conditions in my practice: most of the collagen vascular disorders such as fibromyalgia, lupus, rheumatoid arthritis, etc.; both thyroid autoimmune diseases--Hashimoto's and Graves' disease (with the latter it can help aid establishing remission); SIBO and inflammatory bowel diseases such as Crohn's and ulcerative colitis.

Most patients handle LDN without problem, especially with the titration we do initially. The most common side effects are vivid dreams, which for most go away after a few days, and at times feeling sleepy the next day. If that is happening I move when they take LDN and that can help. I'd say maybe 5-7% of patients do not handle it well.

Overall, outcomes are typically very positive, although, to be honest, I am mixing the LDN with a complex protocol of naturopathic care. People have less pain, antibodies go down, they can function better, their disease is more manageable. Many patients want to stay on it and never go off, which is fine. I find LDN to be a valuable tool as a naturopathic modality in care for patients.

Darin Ingels, ND, FAAEM, FMAPS, USA

I have been using low dose naltrexone in my practice over the past 24 years and find it a valuable tool in the management of pain, autoimmune disease, Lyme disease, autism and more.

I first learned about LDN shortly after my residency training, from a local compounding pharmacist who lectured at a conference I was attending. Given the research and excellent safety profile for children and adults, I started using it in my clinical practice. The majority of my patients find it helps control their symptoms, often even within the first few weeks of using it. As a naturopathic doctor, I am always looking for safe, effective therapies that help in the treatment of chronic illness and LDN has become one of my go-to treatments of choice.

I have treated various illnesses with LDN, but use it primarily in my patients with Lyme disease, autoimmune disease and autism. Since all of these conditions have some element of inflammation, I find that LDN can play an important role in controlling the inflammation and helping patients enjoy a better quality of life. I've seen patients experience less pain, better mobility, deeper sleep, improved mood and overall better sense of well-being. For anyone living with a chronic illness, these are huge wins.

I and my patients appreciate that LDN is also cost-effective, unlike many other more expensive therapies that often come with greater side effects. For anyone dealing with chronic, complex illness, LDN is definitely worth a try.

Samantha Lebsock, PharmD, USA

I was introduced to low dose naltrexone in 2014 when I started out as a compounding pharmacist. The pharmacy has been compounding low dose naltrexone for over 15 years. I was so intrigued by all the different indications that people were using this one drug for.

In 2016, I attended my first LDN conference, where I met Linda Elsegood from the LDN Research Trust. I found myself fascinated with the research and became one of the first LDN Specialists endorsed by the Trust. My passion for LDN continues to grow, as our provider reach expands. We ship LDN across the country, servicing patients in all states. Our scored tablets offer the customization essential for convenient LDN dose titration, a fundamental step for any therapeutic need.

Cultivating a strong base within the integrative and functional medicine space, our LDN prescriptions assist patients combating autoimmune conditions such as Hashimoto's disease and chronic pain conditions, like fibromyalgia. Decreasing flares and fatigue can greatly improve a patient's quality of life.

Our weight management patients aim to benefit from LDN's effect on cravings and appetite regulation in the brain, resulting in meaningful strides towards improved health. More recently, our pharmacy began compounding ultra-low dose naltrexone (ULDN) in a scored, 2 mcg tablet designed to support chronic pain patients on opioid therapy.

My favorite thing about this one drug is how it has improved so many different types of patients' quality of life.

P. McLaughlin, MS, DEd, USA

The observation that low doses of naltrexone inhibited cell proliferation was first observed in our laboratory and published in the Journal of Science in 1983. We were surprised by the observation that more naltrexone was not better for treatment of cancer cells growing in culture and in nude mice. There seemed to be a biphasic response – low dosages inhibited growth; higher dosages accelerated growth.

Since the 1980s, we have studied this phenomenon as it relates to causes and treatment of diseases. We have identified, isolated, and cloned (and validated) the receptor that low dose naltrexone binds in order to inhibit growth. This system - the opioid growth factor – opioid growth factor receptor (OGF-OGFr) regulatory axis – is present in most tissues and species.

After the term "LDN" was coined for the low dosages of naltrexone that intermittently bind to the OGFr, research exploded and many other clinicians and basic scientists began studying and/or prescribing LDN.

Today, LDN is used for treatment of fatigue, fibromyalgia, autoimmune diseases, and pain with good results. We have even heard of LDN successfully being prescribed for treatment of pets. At this time, usage of LDN is based on word-of-mouth success stories as it is still not approved by the FDA.

My suggestion for folks wanting to obtain LDN is to use the websites (there are many) for finding a physician and educating her/him on the benefits of LDN. To date, there are few side effects and many clinical rewards.

Stephen Anderson, RPh, USA

As a compounding pharmacy, we are in a tremendous position to share the significant potential and impact that properly prescribed LDN creates in peoples' lives.

We have compounded LDN off and on for over 25 years; but to a more substantial degree in the last four years. After attending the LDN Research Trust international conference in 2019, our pharmacists made an important decision to expand our clinical understanding of LDN to facilitate our patient consultation abilities and strengthen our collaboration with our prescribing physicians.

Our pharmacists are heavily involved in the consultations/follow-ups of our patients' LDN therapy, assisting our medical providers in the critically important aspect of personalizing their patients' LDN prescription to the most effective dose.

This focused, individualized approach to dosing LDN has resulted in thousands of patients experiencing more successful clinical outcomes across the whole health spectrum.

Patients and providers alike have been exceptionally pleased with the positive mental/brain health outcomes that properly-dosed LDN has provided; it definitely is an unexpected bonus on top of their clinical improvements in the autoimmune, inflammatory and pain realms.

Terry Wingo, RPh, USA

My first call for LDN was in 2004; today we compound LDN for several hundred patients. I've been a community pharmacist for 48 years and have had a compounding-only practice for 24 years.

No other single agent in my career has provided the impact on patients that appropriately dosed and prepared LDN has. We work from a functional/wellness perspective and particularly like that, rather than managing symptoms, LDN helps to rebalance and reset the patient's own biochemical processes. It provides practically universal benefit with chronically-ill patients, so with appropriate counsel I have few reservations in recommending this therapy.

Just one of the many memorable patients that we have worked with was an MS patient who was significantly impaired, unable to participate in basic activities of life. During a wellness consultation we suggested a trial with LDN. Her MS specialist wasn't willing to prescribe, but she was motivated and found another prescriber. She reported after six weeks that 80% of her pain was gone. She went back to her specialist and asked that they repeat her imaging, and found that the most recent lesion was no longer evident. She now encourages other MS patients to explore LDN to improve their own quality of life.

Apelles Econs, MD, UK

As a medical consultant dealing with people with most chronic conditions, I first became aware of LDN in 2012, when I realised that it has been found to help people with MS to reduce muscle spasm. Since then more clinical studies have shown benefits in a wide range of autoimmune disorders such as inflammatory arthritis, inflammatory bowel disease, different types of cancer, atopic eczema, autism spectrum disorder and so on.

The attraction of LDN lies in three main areas:

• Safety is exceptional (doesn't act like a "drug")
• Its indications apply to many chronic disorders which lack options for effective management
• Some patients do not seem to need any other interventions to stay in good health, long term.

I have found LDN helpful to a variable degree in 75% of patients. I prescribe it when effective benefits continue while taking it and benefits dissipate when it is stopped. It is tolerated well, even by chemically-sensitive people.

In my practice, the two most prescribed forms are the sublingual drops and the capsules. The daily dose varies from 0.5-10 mg daily.

Due to its being combined with other treatments in my clinics, it is difficult to objectively assess its influence on specific investigations.

One of the most spectacular examples of LDN-related benefits is a case of a 73-year-old female patient with cutaneous lupus eythematosus which reversed within a few weeks during a course of LDN.

Neel Mehta, MD, USA

I discovered low dose naltrexone in 2017 through the work of some colleagues and learned about its potential to impact pain. I tried it, had some successes, then some failures, but what it did was spark a curiosity for this miracle molecule.

Fast forward to 2023, I have over 700 patients actively using the medication. I have heard patients share stories about its life-changing benefit, surprised at how many other treatments had previously failed, and why it isn't more publicly known.

I have had success in treating all types of pain including myofascial pain, Ehlers-Danlos syndrome, hypermobility, diabetic neuropathy, fibromyalgia, and trigeminal neuralgia.

Together, with Linda Elsegood, I have been fortunate to educate my peers. I have lectured more than 25 times on the use of the medication, including at Cornell, Johns Hopkins, Montefiore, New York University, Yale, and University of Vermont. I have given numerous conference talks, and have educated over 200 fellows of pain management about LDN's potential.

I applaud the efforts here and hope to continue to partner with the LDN Research Trust.

Samyadev Datta, MD, FRCA(Eng), USA

I heard about LDN from James Broatch of the RSDSA about 12 to 14 years ago. I started prescribing LDN almost immediately.

I was starting my patients at 1.5 mg to begin with but have since modified my practice and am willing to start at 0.5 mg and explain to the patients that it may take more time, but it is more likely to be successful.

The average dose across the board is about 5 mg. The highest dose we have a patient on is 7 mg.

About 70-75% of our patients have a positive response, though not everyone responds very well.

I do not do any testing to evaluate for pain management, but do enquire about their functional status and patient self-reporting.

Case Study: ES is an attorney who had come to the office for possible ketamine infusions for management of bilateral lower extremity CRPS. She had given up her law practice as she could not stand on her feet due to pain. She was studying to become a priest when she came to our office. I suggested LDN.

Over the next few months we got her pain under control with LDN and occasional oral ketamine. She did complete her study of theology, but as she was doing so well, has gone back to practicing law full time. She reports that it has changed her life completely.

Dr Lucia Batty, FRCP, FFOM, AFMCP, DipIBLM, UK

I have worked in the NHS for almost three decades and observed the undesired side effects that pharmaceutical drugs commonly have on patients. With this in mind I am delighted to have discovered low dose naltrexone (LDN).

About six years ago I expanded my conventional medical practice by training in Functional Medicine (FM) and consolidated this post-pandemic with accreditation in Lifestyle Medicine (LM). These are two very different, yet complementary approaches to western medicine. FM seeks to answer the question "why" and investigates underlying causes that contribute to and fuel chronic medical conditions. LM is an evidence-based medical specialty, designed to prevent, stabilise, and where possible, reverse lifestyle diseases that includes diabetes, cardiovascular diseases and obesity and metabolic syndrome. It achieves this through the application of key LM pillars - healthier eating, staying active, better sleep, improved social connections, mental health and resilience and reducing harmful substance use.

I first heard about LDN from a distinguished functional medicine physician Dr Pam Smith, who has been successfully using it in her practice. I subsequently embarked on my own research journey of three years, studying and understanding how LDN works and how it can complement overall management of myriad health conditions. These could range from inflammatory autoimmune diseases (such as Crohn's disease and thyroid disorders), to mood, anxiety and depressive disorders, through to premenstrual syndrome and headaches, chronic pain and skin problems. In my experience over the past few years,

LDN appears to be effective and very well tolerated with minimal side effects. Only temporary side effects have been experienced, with the consideration that it can make no difference, as cited at an LDN conference in 2022. It certainly seems to improve quality of life in conditions such as rheumatoid arthritis, SLE, psoriasis, complex eczema, PTSD, anxiety and depression, sleep disorder, pelvic inflammatory disease and long COVID syndrome. It is especially useful in post viral chronic fatigue syndrome (an energy metabolism deficiency) and fibromyalgia or ME, which in addition to impaired energy metabolism involves inflammatory processes.

Unfortunately, despite growing evidence and successful use for over two decades in the United States and many other countries around the world, it remains unlicensed (for many valid reasons) and needs to be ordered on private prescription and compounded in specialised pharmacies. Only some of the GPs and UK NHS specialists in e.g. rheumatology and chronic pain clinics, are prescribing it.

LDN is a pharmacological medication, but up to 10 times weaker (approximately 4.5 mg) than the dose of naltrexone (50-100mg) used in psychiatry for the management of opioid dependence and treatment of alcohol use disorders. It has a short half-life, around 4-6 hours, and works in synergy and harmony with the body, ideally, during the night when sleeping. It seems to have a lasting impact for about 12 hours afterwards. In my practice, the majority of patients I see start low or very low, and build up their doses from about 0.5 mg to 4.5 mg over the period of 4-6 weeks.

LDN appears to work on multiple pathways. Firstly, it partially blocks and stimulates opioid receptors that promote increased endogenous production of the body's own hormones and neurotransmitters, including serotonin (happy hormone) and melatonin (sleep hormone and a very important immunomodulator) and dopamine (reward hormone, gives energy and helps brain solve problems). It has promising potential due to observing its function even as a potent pain-relieving agent used in the management of chronic neuropathic pain. It also has a fascinating function in the way it blocks the Toll-like (TLR-4) receptors and may prevent viruses, bacteria and other microbes from binding on immunological receptors throughout the body. In this respect it may reduce the severity of an immunological reaction, which, for example, in the case of COVID infection, is called a cytokine storm. It competes with a virus and may not allow the virus to cause widespread complex release of multiple chemicals that lead to more severe disease, which was observed and published in acute COVID infection.

LDN has been a surprisingly safe and effective measure for many of my patients. I work in close collaboration with one of the specialist pharmacies in London that compounds LDN. The LDN form of preparation can be personalised i.e., for those with bile acid malabsorption or for those sensitive or allergic to excipients such as silica gel or methyl cellulose. Alternatives can be always be found, as I experienced through effective collaboration between the pharmacy and patients.

I believe that response and hopefully progress with LDN should be objectively monitored. I tend to use various strategies to monitor its impact in addition to individual observations and perceptions. For example, for mental health, we would use the PHQ-9 (for depression), GAD-7 (for anxiety) questionnaire and the PSS (Perceived Stress Scale) assessments. For long COVID syndrome we would use the quality-of-life assessment and visual analogue scale (VAS) for pain self-assessment, whilst for work the work and social adjustment scale (WSAS) would be used in occupational health and wellbeing evaluation. For inflammatory processes and oncology, we would use various inflammatory markers that range from common ones such as ESR, CRP, white cell count and platelets, to more advanced earlier markers of inflammation that could include raised insulin, leptin, LDL, triglycerides and even measure of the extra extracellular water. We can now undertake state-of-the-art wellness screening to identify if the lymphatic system is sluggish with enlarged lymph nodes, using the Multiscan via the Bodyscan360 company. I also noted that patients like to track their own progress. In this regard, on a few occasions some of my patients admitted to stopping LDN without advising me as their practitioner to understand if their system had reset itself and if their bodies have fully restored function they had previously enjoyed. In most circumstances they found that functional capacity, energy and enjoyment was reduced when they came off it. Some patients were very resourceful, using impressive, self-made digital tracking tools.

I have had several patients who have improved target function, for example in case of long COVID syndrome, Hashimoto's thyroiditis, Crohn's disease, type II diabetes, SLE and RA as well as post malignancy and some with full recovery or remission – usually on combination of LDN on top of their own treatment and nutritional and lifestyle interventions.

In my practice I integrate preventive, lifestyle, functional, nutritional and conventional medicine in combination to provide a truly holistic approach to each patient. Patient feedback to LDN has been surprisingly positive and I hope to be able to help many more people in the future.

PAIN CONDITIONS

ARTHRITIS

Elizabeth, USA – Psoriatic Arthritis

I take LDN for psoriatic arthritis (PsA). I was diagnosed with eczema when I was not even one-year-old and later developed psoriasis. I started having symptoms of psoriatic arthritis in my early twenties but I did not have health insurance and was unable to see a specialist. I brought up my concerns to a couple of doctors but they brushed me off by saying they didn't think I had PsA or that I was too young to have it.

Over the years my symptoms would fluctuate; at the worst I had psoriasis completely covering my scalp like a helmet and it was on over 60% of the rest of body, a couple of my fingers and toes were swollen and deformed, and both of my knees were severely swollen, plus I had stomach issues. I hobbled down the hallway at work and sometimes on my days off I was in so much pain in my ankles that I could only crawl at my house. Running around to play with my kids was completely out of the question.

The symptoms would seem to come and go without rhyme or reason. At one point my knees were so swollen that I went to urgent care where the doctor drained off some of the fluid. He said he had never drained so much fluid off of someone's knees and was concerned about draining it all completely. He gave me a steroid shot (the swelling was completely back within one week) and he suggested I go on an anti-inflammatory diet. I had never heard of that but I researched it and changed my diet, which resulted in some improvement of my symptoms, but my knees were permanently swollen like water balloons.

I obtained health insurance when I was 37 and saw a rheumatologist who then officially diagnosed me with psoriatic arthritis. He immediately injected steroids into my knees and put me on methotrexate (MTX), which is a pretty serious drug that required a prescription for daily folic acid and frequent blood testing to check my liver function. My symptoms almost disappeared immediately, but within a couple of months I developed a severe cough. I didn't realize it was related to the MTX because I didn't see that listed anywhere as an adverse symptom. But I was able to find a functional nurse practitioner (NP) who told me that the MTX was basically eating away at the lining of my mucosa and he told me about LDN.

I called my rheumatologist about my cough and he told me to stop methotrexate immediately and he wanted to put me on steroids and biologics. I talked with him about LDN but he made fun of it and said it wasn't FDA approved, and why would I want to try something like that? But what he had prescribed almost destroyed me from the inside out and I wanted to do something that was better for my body, so I told my functional NP that I was ready to start LDN and he wrote me a prescription that day. I was happy to find the only compounding pharmacy in my state that made LDN was located ten miles from my house. I started it immediately.

The NP told me that it would take about three months before the LDN started to work. My symptoms came back during the time that I was off of MTX and just starting LDN but they were never as severe as before. Mostly, my knees were swollen. But within three months of beginning LDN my symptoms began to improve - the swelling in my knees went down and my pain decreased. It took longer for the psoriasis to fade.

I started LDN in August of 2021 at 1.5 mg. I worked up to 4.5 mg within a couple of months and have stayed on that dosage without fluctuation for nearly two years. I try to eat foods in the most natural state possible, but even when I don't, the symptoms don't come back like they had in the past.

I do not experience any side effects while taking LDN. I take it every evening before bed. I also take one prescription medication for low thyroid and some vitamin supplements.

All of my symptoms are gone! I can see bones in my knees again! I didn't think I would ever again see those! My knees are no longer swollen, my joints don't hurt, I can race (and almost beat) my pre-teen, and the psoriasis is GONE! I exercise multiple times a week (cardio and lifting weights) and am very active. When I walk up the stairs and realize I can do it without pain, I am almost in shock, even though it's been this way for almost two years now. It is a miracle.

I don't personally know anyone who takes LDN, so finding the social media group was such a huge encouragement for me when I was first starting out and had so many questions. I am so thankful for medical people who are finding less harmful ways of treating illness. I am also grateful for people who are willing to share their experiences and bring encouragement to those of us who have been discouraged for years and defeated by the health care system and/or our own bodies. I'm forever grateful - my quality of life has radically improved in ways I wasn't sure was even possible anymore.

Barbara, USA – Rheumatoid Arthritis

I had a very aggressive form of rheumatoid arthritis; I was in so much pain for a very long time. My life was unbearable and no amount of medication helped me except maybe with the exception of high doses of prednisone, which helped a little but the side effects just added to my distress. The weight gain didn't help at all, my joints didn't need extra weight to carry. I had insomnia, mood swings – though whether they were a side effect of the prednisone or my general low mood with all the pain or not I don't know. Other medication I tried was methotrexate, that made me so sick and fatigued even more, I tolerated that for about 3 months before deciding that life was miserable enough without adding to it. Plaquenil wasn't as bad but didn't help at all, the pain and inflammation were still the same, even after many months. I was offered biologics but I'd read some horrific reviews of those, particularly infliximab – which my rheumatologist wanted to prescribe alongside methotrexate – I figured I'd rather just have the problems I was dealing with rather than add to them with toxic drugs.

I was only in my early forties and I was pretty sure I was going to die, in fact, on many occasions, death would have been welcome rather than suffer the intolerable pain and exhaustion, coupled with failed medications which made me realise that the so-called specialists couldn't help me at all. Whatever they did just seemed to add new issues on top of the distress of my original symptoms.

My daughter was always researching, she looks into everything, and on one such search she came across low dose naltrexone (LDN). It took us a while but we eventually found a rheumatologist who agreed to prescribe it, he said that the worst it could do was nothing but there was a high chance that it would help. I didn't want to get my hopes up, I'd been disappointed so many times but, as my daughter said, there appeared to be very few side effects with LDN, and then nothing like the awful side effects I'd had with other drugs. I'd stopped the prednisone a few months before starting LDN, I stopped that because I hated looking in mirrors and seeing my "moon face".

I started LDN just short of two years ago. I remember starting on a really low dose, something like 1 mg, and then increasing as and when I felt it would be okay. I increased to 4.5 mg within a month – I didn't have a problem with it at all! I was sleeping better after the first week. My daughter and husband commented on my better moods, I wasn't nearly so miserable though I still had pain during that month. I did feel better in myself that first month – despite the continuing pain, which was rather odd – perhaps because I was actually getting some sleep.

Day by day I seemed able to do more of the things I used to do. Even getting dressed was no longer a prolonged agonising chore. By three months I was gradually realising that I was moving better and had less pain and the swelling on my hands had subsided quite a lot. It just got better and better. And I lost some of the prednisone weight - that made a huge difference to me mentally and physically.

Now I can do all the things you would expect a 48-year-old woman to do – you wouldn't think there was anything wrong with me at all! LDN is an absolute life saver!

I have to say I am so disappointed in the health services for allowing people to suffer for so long when this simple cheap drug has been around for so many years. I have a life now because of LDN whereas as all I had before was a miserable existence. I am so grateful to my daughter for her relentless researching and for the one rheumatologist who was interested enough in actually helping people to acquaint himself with something other than what's laughingly called "standard care".

Averil, Australia - Polymyalgia and Ankylosing Spondylitis

I started LDN when I developed PMR (polymyalgia rheumatica). The inflammation of my muscles made it difficult to turn over in bed and walk. The only medication offered was steroids which I refused due to side effects.

Eventually I got my GP to write me a prescription for LDN. She was hesitant as she had only 50 mg dose information on her computer and had no knowledge of naltrexone's use in low doses like 4.5 mg. I started at 0.5 mg and slowly worked up.

I had been studying LDN because I have a daughter with AS (ankylosing spondylitis). I started LDN when diagnosed with PMR and was pain and stiffness-free within weeks! I was later diagnosed with non-small cell lung cancer and nodes in my lung. I continued taking LDN during treatment, with oncologist approval, and he was convinced it aided the treatment.

My daughter with AS had chronic sinusitis and costochondritis; she started LDN and both conditions were resolved and never returned. I have not had a cold or flu or respiratory problem since starting LDN three years ago!

Lili, Denmark - Psoriatic Arthritis

I spoke to Linda Elsegood years ago about my journey with LDN. My interview with Linda can be found here https://www.youtube.com/watch?v=jycsG4cWgLY

It is a pleasure for me to continue my story here.

I was diagnosed with psoriatic arthritis (PsA) around 2008 and my rheumatologist medicated me with methotrexate and at that time it did help, but it also gave me a lot of side effects such as unstable blood sugar, bad liver figures if I came above 12 mg/week and many infections. I decided to stop and things went well until 2015.

In the autumn of 2015, it began again and what a blow, the pain was bad, very bad. When I went to bed my feet and body were burning, I hardly slept for several months, the rheumatologists prescribed me methotrexate and prednisolone again, with no effect apart from my blood sugar going berserk. No pain relief whatsoever.

Then I started to research on the internet and LDN popped up; I did a lot of research. It sounded too good to be true, like a bad advertisement, but I asked my GP if he would prescribe it and he agreed.

I started on the 23rd of September 2016 at 9 am, on 0.75 mg and had a good result from day one. My body relaxed, the brain fog vanished, and my feet and body did not go on fire when I went to bed. My PsA had a flare at Christmas time. That was a blow but I continued my LDN journey and in the summer 2017 I began to feel "normal" on 4.5 mg daily, and today on 7 mg my PSA only flares in spring and autumn, when the weather changes.

I have been supported a lot in a Danish LDN group, as my GP had no idea of what to do with LDN, and I studied the LDN Research Trust website as well. I am so grateful for all the information I have had from both sources and am doing my best to tell people about LDN everywhere, but it is a hard job, almost everyone seems to think that it is too good to be true, even though I myself am proof of the efficacy of LDN.

I would probably have been disabled today without LDN and I have not visited a rheumatologist since I started on LDN as they refuse to prescribe it. Many Danish GPs do the same as they consider LDN to be addictive or sort of LSD. Ignorance is very hard to fight, unfortunately.

I give thanks to the LDN Research Trust and my support group for informing me about LDN. I am most grateful.

Anette, Denmark - Psoriatic Arthritis and Back Pain

My name is Anette Møberg, I am 56 years old and a trained physiotherapist.

I have, for approximately 35 years, had back problems and had 30-plus disc herniations/reprolapses. I have osteoarthritis and inflammation in the entire spine, several pinched nerves and also spinal stenosis in several places. Since 2012, I have also suffered from severe psoriatic arthritis, which prevented me from attending my physiotherapy clinic.

Over the years, I have been on countless preparations for both pain and psoriatic arthritis, including methotrexate, biological drugs, antidepressants and opioids. Nothing had a remarkable effect but gave many unpleasant side effects.

In the summer of 2015, I was about to give up due to severe pain, side effects, fatigue, etc., and I was assigned to a pain clinic. They offered LDN. LDN was very new in Denmark at this time, and there were only a few hundred people taking it. I said yes thanks, not knowing what LDN was.

From day one my arthritis calmed down, I had more energy and the fatigue disappeared. I could think again! I had some side effects in the form of vivid dreams, a little headache and nausea, but it went away in a few days. I didn't get complete pain relief immediately, but everything else was enough for me - I was satisfied.

Four and a half months after starting I woke up one morning and was pain free and have been since. One hundred percent pain free and I haven't had a single flare-up in the psoriatic arthritis since the start.

Deeply impressed and interested, I thoroughly familiarized myself with LDN's working mechanisms, and we LDN users here in Denmark met in a social media group where we exchanged experiences. Several doctors joined the group and the spread of knowledge of LDN had begun.

I started giving lectures about LDN, and when the Danish Society for Anaesthesiology and Intensive Medicine asked me to give a lecture at their annual meeting, I knew that in Denmark we had to have an LDN association, so that knowledge of LDN could be spread much more.

The LDN Association is now four and a half years old and we

have a good collaboration with pharmacists, doctors and other patient associations. We create material for both users and healthcare professionals and participate in various conferences.

We now have over 25,000 users in Denmark. All public pain clinics offer LDN.

We are so lucky here in Denmark to have MD. Karin Due Bruun, who has done three research projects in LDN for fibromyalgia, which also means that more general practitioners dare to use LDN, even if they don't know it very well.

Our goal with the LDN Association is to have LDN recognized on an equal footing with all other preparations for pain, autoimmune diseases, cancer etc.

Victoria, USA – Rheumatoid Arthritis

I began having undiagnosed RA symptoms when I was 18 but was not officially diagnosed by a rheumatologist until I was 25. Due to the RA, along with genetically very loose/flexible tendons, I would have horrible pain in my shoulders periodically. I attempted the traditional medications that rheumatologists prescribe, but none of them worked, and the side effects made me feel worse. I had more success with acupuncture and herbs for a few years, but then even that wasn't having the same results I had come to expect.

I started to have issues with my hands and waking up with them feeling like my tendons were "frozen" and I couldn't fully open them for 20-30 minutes. Finally, when I was 31, a co-worker recommended I try her functional medicine doctor. I was beyond impressed – I'd finally found a doctor who would look at everything! She re-did blood work and reconfirmed my RA diagnosis and current levels.

She recommended I try LDN and warned me of some of the potential minimal side effects. I agreed to give it a try and roughly four to five weeks in, only taking 3 mg, I was already seeing a difference. My hands had quit feeling "frozen" in the mornings and overall I had approximately a 50% improvement in the rest of my joint pains. She then increased my dose to 4.5 mg which is where I have stayed for the past two years.

The only side effects I can speak to would be insomnia and vivid dreams. The insomnia resolved itself within three weeks (though I do take a low dose of melatonin nightly) and the vivid dreams continue, but are not disruptive or unpleasant necessarily, just different.

I now regularly look up what conditions LDN may assist with and regularly tell people they should consider looking into it. I have averaged only one RA flare a year since I have started LDN, and I can't imagine my life without it.

Terri, USA - Pain and Inflammation

I take LDN for pain and inflammation, with bone-on-bone pain in my hip. I noticed symptoms years ago, getting steadily worse with time. My life was extremely difficult with pain upon standing, sitting, laying down, even trying to sleep.

I will eventually have surgery to restore structure and function, but in the meantime I was only taking Advil and herbal medications. Nothing was really working until my doctor recommended LDN.

I started taking LDN in January 2023 at 1 mg and it made a difference immediately! The pain relief was astounding, literally two days in! Upon increasing to 2 mg I experienced amazing results! However, increasing to a higher dose than that made me feel funky, creating vivid dreams, and feelings of wooziness. I titrated slowly, 1 mg at a time, but when I increased to 3 mg, and then 4 mg, both doses made me feel hungover, foggy and groggy. I'm happy to say that 2 mg is my optimal feel-good dose.

I still have a little trouble sleeping, but sleep is better than it was. LDN is the only medication I'm using now, and I'm able to move and function in my daily life without being limited by excruciating and debilitating pain. I'm even considering cancelling or postponing my surgery!

As I wait for my surgery date, I am able to maintain independence with most of my activities, especially playing with my grandson, which is the most important thing to me.

Also, we just moved, and I was able to pack my home, carry heavy boxes down two long flights of stairs, and up a long flight into our new home, without any challenges or pain. That's nothing short of a miracle! Thank goodness for LDN.

Paula, UK - Drug Induced Autoimmune Arthritis

It was May 2002, I was 38 with two teenagers and a four-year-old and a six-year-old. I thought it would be a good idea to stop smoking and get healthier – though I wasn't in bad health, there was nothing wrong with me. The NHS was offering smoking cessation courses and I was prescribed Zyban (bupropion hydrochloride, Wellbutrin) through them. The course of Zyban was to last two months; I stopped taking it in less than three weeks. By day three I didn't want to smoke any more, amazing stuff but I also didn't feel "right" on it. By week two I had a horrible pain out of nowhere in my right ankle, by week three the ankle was terribly swollen and hot and I could barely put it down - or pick it up - or sleep because the weight of the sheet on my ankle was unbearable, and this continued for the next 13 years. The doctors naturally said that it *couldn't possibly* be caused by Zyban, though there are now other cases of this online – though "rare" of course, they're always going to be rare if they're not reported and doctors continue to dismiss their patients experiences as "coincidences."

I tried all manner of things, acupuncture, herbs, ice/heat, nothing eased it. I had x-rays that showed nothing. It took two years to get my first rheumatologist and he could barely be bothered to speak. He diagnosed "mono-arthritis" and put me on sulfasalazine for a couple of years which did nothing much except possibly cause more joint pain and random rashes. And he put me on Vioxx which also did very little.

I got a new rheumatologist around 2006/7, he was a nice bloke, friendly, had time for his patients but was unfortunately stuck to standard treatments, whether they worked or not. He changed the diagnosis to psoriatic arthritis simply because I had developed a rash on my left foot.

He prescribed methotrexate, Solpadol 30/500 mg (codeine/paracetamol) and Arcoxia, as Vioxx had been withdrawn due to serious adverse events. I slowly declined mentally and physically, the rash drove me nuts and I had frequent flare-ups of the arthritis which caused a great deal of pain and many sleepless nights. As time went on and the methotrexate dosage increased because it wasn't helping, I started to sleep at the drop of a hat, sometimes falling asleep at my desk at work. Hard going when you have a business to run. It crossed my fuddled brain occasionally that it seemed silly taking these drugs when I was still having pain like I was; there were still lots of days where I couldn't walk at all and the other days limping because the pain was always present. It just depended on where it was as to whether I could walk or not. The pain moved around my ankle, heel/Achilles tendon and foot. Sometimes I also had cortisone injections into the joint so that I could have a "pain holiday." They were okay but still didn't totally eradicate the pain – while the cortisone damaged my cartilage and killed off nearby bone of course (MRI confirmed in 2015).

Then early in 2014 I had a particularly bad flare while away from home. This left me almost breathless with pain, pain that would not lessen regardless of the amount I overdosed on Arcoxia or Solpadol 30/500. That was the last straw for me. I started to read everything I could on autoimmune diseases, methotrexate and anti-inflammatory diets.

I have significant damage to the talar navicular joint in my right ankle. For at least five years I'd been on a drug believing it to be stopping damage when it wasn't doing anything of the sort. In fact it wasn't even positively modifying the symptoms – if anything it was making things worse. The rash was spreading, the pain was bad most days, I had a constant limp when I could actually walk. My right knee was turning inward because of the way I was walking. My right hip ached. And all the while I had chronic inflammation. More annoying still, I suffered constant fatigue, brain fog, hair loss, weight loss and, naturally, depression. I found plenty of other people reporting the same adverse effects from methotrexate. All that misery and zero benefit. Twice, while on methotrexate, 25 mg dose once a week, I had flares in my ankle, shoulder, elbow and wrist – that was frightening.

I set about eliminating all processed junk food from my diet. I ate blended fruits and raw vegetables for a month, with little meat, I had no appetite, really, anyway – sometimes I ate nothing for days. I bought supplements that were anti-inflammatory. And I threw all my medications away, accept the pain killers.

My last dose of methotrexate was on 8th July 2014. At that time I could barely walk, uneven ground was an excruciating experience, a pebble could cause intense shooting pains up my leg. "Coincidentally," according to my rheumatologist, my inflammation markers went down significantly and my liver function was much better once I'd thrown methotrexate in the bin.

I put Canesten on the rash on my left foot – within four days it was clearing up. I didn't have psoriasis to begin with and it was likely a long long fungal infection but nobody checked that. Psoriasis was "assumed" because it was convenient.

After a few months of scrapping all the drugs and changing my diet the inflammation in my ankle and foot had reduced by about half. The pain I did have was tolerable – a mere dull ache compared to what I'd been used to. A different diet had a much better effect than the "DMARD" methotrexate – and yet no medical professional ever suggested a change in diet. I was still taking Solpadol at this stage because I needed pain relief, though not as often.

My rheumatologist was unhappy that I'd scrapped his drugs but then he requested an MRI, the outcome being a referral to a foot and ankle surgeon. The surgeon wanted to fuse my ankle in two places, I said no to that, not until I can't walk at all. Surgery wasn't going to address the actual problem, the drug induced autoimmune issue would continue regardless, probably in some other joints. He offered me biologic drugs, no chance. My faith in the NHS by this time was below nil; now doctors appeared to me to be a danger I should avoid wherever possible.

Then, in 2015, I was watching Dr. John Bergman, a chiropractor and holistic doctor, on YouTube. He was doing one of his talks on inflammation. He said "I don't usually suggest pharmaceutical drugs but low dose naltrexone is one of the good ones," or words to that effect. I started researching it.

Most of my research was done on the LDN Research Trust website. Vast amounts of information about LDN use in all manner of autoimmune diseases. I'd also read what the naysayers had to say:

"Snake oil, nothing treats that many different illnesses" was a common one but with a little research you soon realise that all those different illnesses are caused by the same thing basically – immune system dysfunction. LDN was worth a try because the side-effect profile looked really good and reading other peoples' experiences, the real evidence of any drug, it didn't look like much of a risk.

I finally got my private prescription for LDN on 5th May 2015. I started on 1 mg and was to increase the dose weekly by 0.5 mg but I got to 4.5 mg before the end of two weeks. By the end of May I had zero inflammation in my ankle and foot, all the inflammation that had been damaging me for 13 years had gone. I could see my ankle bones again! The pain started to wane away within a fortnight and I had more range of motion and I could walk normally. Running isn't possible because the damage I've suffered from years of what I can only call neglect by my "healthcare providers". I can overdo it and cause some pain and little flares but recovery is generally overnight, not days or weeks on end.

My GP refused to even listen or look at the information I'd taken for him about LDN. Of course, I was no longer taking methotrexate, Arcoxia or Solpadol and I no longer wanted cortisone injections – less drugs don't appear to be the goal, neither does anything that might give a person some quality of life.

LDN has given me my life back. I'm angry that my doctors aren't remotely interested in why I no longer require four drugs, for the last eight years, including pain relief, for a degenerative disease that's clearly stopped degenerating. It's also more than annoying that this safe and effective drug has been there all that time and I wasn't offered it as a first line treatment. I only take LDN now, nothing else, I don't even need pain killers any more.

Now I walk my dogs three times a day, I walk into town rather than drive – because I can. I can do all the things I could do before that stupid decision to stop smoking using Zyban, except run of course, the damage doesn't allow for running.

I had no side effects with LDN, not even vivid dreams. My depression lifted within the first two weeks. I had hope again because without

LDN I'd be in a wheelchair now, as promised by my rheumatologist, "You'll be in a wheelchair within the next few years" he said, and that was while I was destroying my life with his drugs. Such was his faith in his own treatments.

LDN is not a cure, though it feels like one. If I stop taking it the disease process will pick up where it left off; it takes about three days without LDN before I feel the pain and stiffness, due to inflammation, creep back in. But while I'm taking LDN I'm absolutely fine, happy, energetic, pain free and clear headed. And I now eat a pretty good normal diet, though no processed garbage.

If you're curious about LDN but hesitant to try it - just go for it. The absolute worst it can do is nothing and there is a very high success rate with LDN for all manner of autoimmune conditions. Just be sure to talk to a qualified LDN specialist who will tell you the best way for you to start for your condition.

Hayley, US – Rheumatoid Arthritis

I first had symptoms seven years ago at the age of 45. It started in my feet and I asked my doctor for help because it was getting very painful.

He sent me for x-rays on my feet and that showed nothing was wrong. He then thought I had a viral infection and put me on a course of antivirals but that did nothing. Then a podiatrist thought my arches were too high so gave me a series of exercises to do and some inserts for my shoes, but they just hurt me more. The exercises became too hard to do because the pain was increasing. I was even told that I must have injured my feet; though I knew I hadn't had any accidents. It was so frustrating because the doctors I'd seen just seemed to think something up and want to treat me with various things but there was no firm diagnosis. I knew I hadn't fallen; I was baffled about how a virus could cause pains in my feet and if I had high arches then it had never been mentioned before or given me any problems.

It took 3 years to get a proper diagnosis. They finally did a rheumatoid factor test and found it was very high. I saw a rheumatologist and she said it was RA. She then prescribed me lots of medications for the pain and inflammation – so then I had all the side effects of those and no let-up in my painful symptoms. I still had pain, inflammation and I had more fatigue than ever and I just felt horrible.

I realised that there was no help at all coming from the standard medical establishment. The pain was spreading to other joints and my future was looking exceedingly dark to my mind. After a few years of that, and realising I needed to help myself, I started to research and joined groups of others suffering from RA, and that's where I first heard about LDN.

I had no side effects at all when I started LDN but I did have symptom relief within three weeks, the swelling going down over the following few months. The pain ebbed away first, and with it the fatigue and then the inflammation. I got rid of all the other prescribed drugs – which in itself improved my quality of life. It was wonderful to be able to move properly again and to be able to stay awake all day, and wonderful to be able to sleep through a night without being jolted by pain as I was drifting off.

I would tell anybody who's thinking about taking LDN to try it, it restored my quality of life, it gave me my life back and for that I'm really grateful. I'm also grateful for all those who share their stories in the support groups online, without them I would never have heard of LDN.

CHRONIC FATIGUE SYNDROME

Alison, USA – Chronic Fatigue Syndrome and Dysautonomia

When I was 30 years old, back in 1992, I suddenly got very sick with symptoms of flu and mono. Weeks and months went by with no answers as all my tests came back negative. I was told it was probably anxiety because I was a young woman who had two children so I was probably stressed out. My symptoms were extreme fatigue, I had to sleep 16 hours a night and take naps in the day when my children were napping or in school. I had nausea, digestive issues, vertigo at times, blood pressure drops, night sweats and day sweats, dizziness, irregular heartbeats and low-grade fevers at times. I was eventually diagnosed with chronic fatigue syndrome and dysautonomia.

I was very bad for a good ten years, mostly housebound. I couldn't do things with my children, take them places or enjoy them. My husband had to do the food shopping on the weekends when he was off from working his 60-hour work weeks. Life was very lonely as I lost friends and even family members; they just couldn't believe I could be that severely sick and doctors wouldn't know how to help me. They thought I was exaggerating or it was all in my head, from some of the remarks I've heard them say. It was a living nightmare. I would tell my husband I felt like I was in a sci-fi movie of a virus that attacked my nervous system.

I tried everything I could do to heal. I did acupuncture, different types of massage therapy, herbs, every type of holistic modality you can think of. We spent a lot of money on these therapies in hopes to get some relief. I would get a little relief at times from certain things but it never lasted. The doctors had no help for me except medication to help the insomnia issue that comes with this nervous system damage from chronic fatigue syndrome and that's what caused dysautonomia. We were financially strapped as I had to stop working and I continued to spend a lot of money on trying new treatments that came along.

Twenty-three years later I was on social media in chronic fatigue and fibromyalgia groups. I would read some talking about this treatment called low dose naltrexone and all the success they were having with it. I didn't want to dive in right away so I would just watch the page for over a year before I would finally do it. I was very sensitive to medications of any type and had lots of allergies to things so I was very apprehensive to try yet another, what I perceived to be, questionable treatment.

After a while I decided to ask my integrative doctor for a prescription for LDN. I was seeing him for a good year at this point and was surprised he hadn't already mention this to me; actually I was very upset about it. He gave me a prescription and wanted me to start at 4.5 mg but after educating myself on patients with chronic fatigue syndrome it seemed like we needed to start at a lower dose than that. I had asked him for a prescription for 0.5 mg.

I started the 0.5 mg and that first night I felt like I had insomnia and some nausea but the next day I had more energy than I've had in a long time, brain fog was lifted a lot and I just felt better all around. I figured "Oh it's probably the placebo effect" so I didn't want to get my hopes up.

After about a week I was still feeling good in the daytime. Although some insomnia was still happening it was worth it. I started being able to do more things and getting out of the house more; I even took a yoga class, which I haven't done in decades. Everybody around me was starting to see the benefits I was having on this treatment. I felt like I was finally starting to get some life back. At times I would clean my house and do the normal things the average person does but I would still relapse if I pushed myself too much. I thought if I went up in dose I would have even better gains. I slowly worked my way up to 3 mg. I actually felt some anxiety at times and I was starting to feel sicker. I stopped LDN for a couple of months so that I can reset my body. I started back at 0.5 mg and that is what I'm currently taking now. I've been on LDN for seven years now and my life is so much better.

I am not cured, I still relapse if I overdo it and I know my energy and stamina is not as good as the average healthy 60-year-old woman but it's so much better than it was. When I was first sick I could rate my life at 1, sometimes a 2, on a scale of 1 to 10. Now I would say I am a 6, sometimes 7 on a scale of 1 to 10, 10 being the average healthy 60-year-old and 0 being dead.

I always prayed for a good safe treatment to come along and never gave up hope, and sure enough it did! LDN has given me some life back and for that I am forever grateful.

Kathy, UK – Chronic Fatigue Syndrome

Thirty years ago I developed chronic bronchitis due to my boss chain smoking in my office at work. I became very ill and was admitted into hospital, and from there my health deteriorated. Life became very very difficult. I had two young daughters and had to give up work due to ill health.

I tried so many treatments, including hyperbaric treatment, numerous supplements, very expensive tablets to enhance mitochondria. I also went to a health clinic in London who were supposed to heal CFS. I had absolutely no positive results. I tried too many medications to list. I tried everything available. Nothing worked until I started LDN.

I heard about LDN from a friend who had CFS. It has truly been a miracle for me after being so unwell for so long. Nothing else worked. I spent thousands seeking a cure. I will forever be grateful for LDN.

I started LDN around November 2021 on the lowest dose and I increased the dose gradually until I found my ideal which is 4 mg per day.

Initially I found that I couldn't sleep so I started taking it in the morning and since then I've slept really well. I have had no other negative side effects.

I started to notice improvements in my condition after around four to six weeks. I was overjoyed that I was at long last getting my life back. The fatigue lifted and I slept well. My GP was delighted at how well I was after many years being so unwell. They had never heard of LDN previously and I was pleased that they asked for more information about it, which I supplied.

I only take thyroxine and LDN now. LDN has been a true miracle. Almost too good to be true. It's given me back my life. This is a truly amazing drug. It should be available on the NHS. It seems so unfair that so many people are suffering yet this amazing drug, LDN, is available. Seems very sad that people are left to suffer, unless you can afford to go privately to obtain it.

What is Chronic Fatigue Syndrome (ME/CFS)?

Chronic fatigue syndrome is a debilitating illness featuring extreme fatigue that cannot be relieved with rest. Along with the fatigue comes muscle pain, joint pain, headaches, post-exertional malaise, and the mental health issues that you would expect with pain and fatigue – anxiety, lack of concentration and depression.

ME (myalgic encephalomyelitis)/CFS are thought to be the same illness, called CFS in the USA from the 1980s and ME in the UK in the 1950s – both names now combine under the umbrella term ME/CFS.

Diagnosis is a process of elimination of other known illnesses; there is no single test to diagnose this horrible illness. There are many people suffering with this illness, the majority being women, who have not been diagnosed.

Treatment consists of pharmaceuticals ranging from pain relievers, non-steroidal anti-inflammatory drugs (NSAIDs), anticonvulsants, antidepressants and narcotics to antiviral and immunomodulatory drugs to relieve symptoms. The side effects of the many drugs just add to the problem.

There are many studies and case reports discussing LDN as an effective treatment for ME/CFS. If this one simple, safe and effective drug can do what all those other drugs often fail to do, without adding unpleasant side effects, then there is nothing to lose from trying it and everything to gain.

FIBROMYALGIA

Kendra, USA – Fibromyalgia and Depression

I have suffered with fibromyalgia since 2017, though it took such a long time and quite a few different drugs, before I had an actual diagnosis that the doctors felt fit my symptoms perfectly. First I was told it was rheumatoid arthritis, then I was tested for Lyme disease, then it was lupus but as time passed, and my symptoms didn't follow those disease paths, it was decided that it was fibromyalgia. Personally, I don't care what it's called, it hurt and it's miserable and I just wanted to get better.

My husband had been to the doctors and he noticed a leaflet on the wall advertising a fibromyalgia support group not far from where we live. I normally dislike group settings but I wanted to not feel so alone, and I was surprised by the support and encouragement I received from the other members. Their sense of humor, despite their suffering, inspired me to no end and I was surprised to see how much better I felt mentally knowing that these good people were there for me and for each other.

We discussed our treatments and how we were doing on them and a couple of the members were on low dose naltrexone. We discussed that a lot because they seemed to be doing so much better than anybody else. Most of us were a little scared to try it; we'd all had bad experiences with new drugs. I was, at that time, on Lyrica and it helped with the pain and it helped with sleep a little too much. I wanted to sleep a lot, which wasn't helpful and fatigue is part of the illness and Lyrica seemed to make that worse. I gained weight while on Lyrica too and I wasn't happy about that.

Several of the other members decided to try LDN too. They could take it alongside their other drugs, so long as they weren't on opiates they were told, except one lady on Cymbalta, she had to stop her Cymbalta first her doctor said. She did manage to do this and was grateful that she'd made that choice. All four of these ladies had benefits from LDN, some more than others but all to a degree that surprised us. This is where I got the courage from to try it.

One of my primary issues, apart from the pain, was my mental outlook. I was scared of what was in my future, what it would hold for me. I suppose it was depression because who isn't going to be depressed when in constant pain and permanently fatigued. My thoughts were sometimes really dark and it took effort to not go down the road those thoughts were wanting to take me.

My rheumatologist had heard of LDN but had never prescribed it. He took some convincing but I presented the cases of the ladies in the group and he eventually agreed. I started on 1 mg and worked up to 4.5 mg over a period of six weeks. And each increase added a new band of colour to my rainbow. I did have some trouble with really vivid dreams, while pleasant, they weren't restful at all but that only lasted about a week or so. Otherwise I suffered no unwanted side effects at all.

I had a gradual decrease in pain after the first month and now I sleep really well and can move so much better. I'm so happy the pain is leaving me; I still have a little but it's more of a nuisance than a spoiler of the day and it's easily controlled with regular pain pills if it gets more than irritating. I've been taking LDN for a year and three months as I write this and my mental outlook is fabulous now, everything is positive and I live like every day is precious – because it is.

Rebecca Peck, APRN, USA - Fibromyalgia

About six years ago, in 2017, I worked as an RN in a local hospital's clinical liaison department. During that time, I met a fibromyalgia patient who shared her positive experience with low dose naltrexone (LDN), igniting my curiosity. Dealing with fibromyalgia myself, I was eager to learn more and made a note of "LDN" for further investigation.

That day, I began my research on LDN. Later, armed with a printed journal article, I approached my PCP, hopeful that LDN could bring relief, but she couldn't prescribe it due to the lack of FDA approval for treating fibromyalgia with LDN.

Undeterred, I spent the next five years searching for a local doctor willing to prescribe LDN. My pain intensified, and I began relying on 30 mg of Vicodin, later transitioning to 30 mg of oxycodone daily to manage the persistent pain.

Struggling with my distant pain management doctor, I sought a local solution. In a pivotal consultation in September 2022, a doctor in my town suggested LDN as a viable alternative, provided I weaned off oxycodone within 30 days.

In October 2022, LDN treatment commenced at 5 mg twice a day. While the start brought some nausea and vomiting, Zofran helped alleviate these initial challenges.

Within a month, the changes were evident - more energy, reduced pain, and a diminished desire for opiates. I transitioned from a bedridden state on oxycodone, unable to endure a six hour shift, to flourishing as a family nurse practitioner. Now, my days encompass 6-7 days a week, 8-12-hour shifts - an inspiring journey from agony to triumph.

For more information on LDN and its use in treating fibromyalgia, a Google search will quickly bring up the LDN Research Trust and many clinical trials showing positive results for LDN and fibromyalgia. There are also many journal articles revealing positive results for LDN for many other autoimmune/inflammatory disease states, as well as mental health conditions.

Karen, Australia – Fibromyalgia

I first noticed symptoms in 2011, I had pain from head to toe and most days I was bed ridden. I virtually had no life as I stopped going out in case someone touched me. I couldn't work, life was miserable. I would be at my doctor's every week hoping that there was something he could give me that would stop the pain, even for just a few days, I was that desperate.

I tried EVERY pain relief my doctor offered me, oxycodone, Targin, tramadol etc., all not very effective, and most would make me feel sick. I was given all sorts of antidepressants; they did absolutely nothing. I honestly lost count of how many different medications I was prescribed.

My mother's friend, from her cancer group, told her about LDN and she told me about it. I then did some research on it and I am so grateful to her because it saved my life.

I presented my own research to my doctor and he had never heard of it before but because he knew the pain I had been going through for years he agreed to write me a prescription. All the information was there to tell him how to prescribe it for a compounding pharmacy.

I started taking LDN in 2015 at 1.5 mg per day and increased steadily until I felt happy at 5 mg. Initially I went through herxing two weeks after starting. I thought I was dying, it was so bad. But worse I felt that LDN wasn't going to work for me. I am so glad I persevered because after about three weeks that's when the miracle happened and I have never looked back. One other side effect, which still happens occasionally, is vivid dreams but they are awesome, I really don't mind those.

I noticed improvement almost immediately, until the herxing started but that passed and left me with nothing but improvements to my quality of life. I now have minimal brain fog and the flare-ups that used to happen every other week are now maybe once every six or eight months and they are nowhere near as bad as they were before. The pain all over is greatly reduced.

The benefits from taking LDN means that I can now live a relatively normal life again. There are still occasional fibro flares and other associated things that go along with fibro, but I'm able to work again and socialize with friends. LDN has been my life saver.

Amy, USA - Fibromyalgia

After years of declining health, at the age of 49, I was losing the strength in my large group muscles, especially my thighs. My GP suggested I had fibromyalgia. My office is on the second floor of a huge building and I couldn't walk up the two flights without putting my hands on my thighs to give them stability. My husband worried that I was going to end up in a wheelchair.

A functional medicine doctor I followed on social media was bringing attention to the use of LDN and the conditions it could help.

At work, I had just been offered to help lead a trip to Israel and I didn't want to miss the opportunity, so I decided to give LDN a try.

Within two weeks, it was as if I was given a new life. By the time I went to Israel, I had the energy that I needed to organize 56 travellers for 9 days and walk 3 to 6 miles a day touring. I can also ride my bike and push mow my lawn, which is on an incline.

I had minimal side effects. No strange dreams. For the first two weeks, I did have an infection that pushed itself out of my body through cysts that formed in my ears, behind my ears and in my neck.

I started at 1 mg and kept increasing by 0.5 mg every week or so. I have stayed at 3.5 mg for many years.

Thankfully, my GP was open to giving me a prescription. Through the years he said that he had several patients on it, but that I was the one who had the most dramatic results. LDN has given me my life back and allowed me to be an active person. I will be 57 years old soon.

Jane, Australia - Fibromyalgia

In July 2015 I went to see a new GP, Dr. B, in NSW Australia. I had had pain all over my body for some time and it was getting worse. There were times when I would be crying at work with the pain and exhaustion of it. I had decided if she couldn't help me I needed to quit work. The pain, alongside "in the red" ANA readings, was increasing. ANA had been abnormal for eight years by then. I had seen a rheumatologist about three years before. She did nothing.

Dr. B put me on 1.5 mg of LDN after diagnosing me with fibromyalgia. Over the next few days the pain started to recede, within three weeks it was 80% gone. Over the next few months it went completely. In July 2016 Dr. B re-tested my ANA. For the first time, in over eight years, it was in the black! No more autoimmune condition. Dr. B was amazed. She had never seen an autoimmune condition reverse.

As the years went on, if a tiny bit of pain surfaces anywhere, I change the dose to less or more depending on how I'm feeling. I've been on 0.5, 1.5, 3 and 4.5 mg. If I go off LDN the pain creeps back over time. So I stay on it, and I rarely get others' colds, flus etc. It has fixed my immune system.

I had no side effects apart from lucid dreams. I slept well on it for a long time, but will say if I have any issues with sleep I switch to mornings for a while. I will never not take it. When Dr. B went on extended leave I had trouble finding a doctor to prescribe it but with perseverance I've always managed to find someone willing. She is back now and happy to keep prescribing it. Here in Australia it costs about $1 AUD a day.

Ina, Australia - Fibromyalgia

I have had fibromyalgia for nine years and it was difficult to get through the day. Even minor activities like taking a shower or walking within the house were a problem on many days. Some days were better and I was able to leave my home but then my anxiety level increased substantially doing so.

Finally, an integrative doctor prescribed LDN. It was a life changer! I started on 0.5 mg and knew from day one that this was good for me. I felt better immediately. I still increased to 2 mg a day and have been on this dose for five years now.

The only side effects were some vivid dreams initially, maybe for a few months, which was more of a surprise than an unpleasant experience.

I still have a day on crutches occasionally but I also have some pain-free days, which was unheard of before. LDN has returned a quality of life that I am very grateful for.

Nichole, USA – Fibromyalgia

I currently take LDN for fibromyalgia. I have chronic widespread pain in my body, particularly my hands. I have a fibromyalgia-type illness that's currently still under-diagnosed formally.

Prior to starting LDN I had sudden onset of body pain, nerve pain, depression, etc. Most doctors gave me SSRIs and SSNRIs, or anti-seizure meds. I was taking three to four medications trying to manage the symptoms but was never successful.

Finally, after doing my own research about LDN for pain management and how it's harmless to try it, I was able to obtain a prescription, paying about 100 dollars every 3 months or so. It was easy for me but I can imagine it's a barrier for those who cannot afford it in the US.

After taking it as directed, going from 1 mg up to now 4.5 mg, my widespread pain and weakness is gone. LDN has been nothing short of a miracle for otherwise disabling pain and fatigue/weakness. I've had no noticeable side effects after being on it for over a year now.

I now take three meds but the other two are for ADHD only. LDN is my only prescription treatment for pain and fatigue.

LDN has given me my life back. I'm young and having to come to terms with having a mysterious chronic pain issue, that doctors couldn't help with, was at times leaving me with suicidal ideations. Since taking LDN I am much happier and can function in normal life.

Eudice, USA – Fibromyalgia

I take LDN for fibromyalgia. I've been on it for many years to help me with pain, insomnia and back problems.

I had to work hard to get a prescription back then. It's easier now. I started at 0.5 mg then went to 1.5 mg and was on that dose for years. Now I take 3 mg.

A few days after I started it, I got a very sharp pain in my back. When I stood up I found that my back, which had been tense and painful, had relaxed and I could stand straight with no pain. Other pains from the fibromyalgia went away also. My doctor now recommends it to his patients.

My sister told me about LDN originally. Her doctor friend told her to try it for her fibromyalgia. His wife had MS and was needing a wheelchair. He researched LDN and gave her it and she was back to playing tennis, no MS symptoms. His son had Crohn's disease and it cleared it up so well that now there's no evidence of him ever having had it on his more recent scans.

I will take LDN till I die. It has given me my life back. I bless the doctor that told my sister about it.

Penny, USA - Fibromyalgia

I've had fibromyalgia for over 25 years. I have had lots of pain issues from that along with arthritis, spinal stenosis, bulging discs, DDD, neuralgia, arthralgia, bone spurs on my shoulders and hips, cluster headaches, insomnia and severe depression. I took Cymbalta, trazodone, Topamax, cyclobenzaprine, oxycodone, gabapentin and low dose naltrexone.

LDN has been a godsend and a total game changer for me. I've had one fibromyalgia flare in three months since I started the LDN. The main thing I feel that LDN has done for me is it's almost totally lifted my severe depression. No more hopelessness. No more feelings of low self-esteem. I've even been able to join a gym again and I've started working out. I don't procrastinate as much anymore.

I started out on 1 mg of LDN for a week then went to 3 mg for three weeks. Went up to 4.5 mg for a month and now I'm on 7.5 mg and that's where I'll stay.

Nothing is a cure all, but I find myself sitting and just smiling because the LDN bumps up your feel-good receptors in the brain and helps block the pain receptors.

I highly recommend you give it a try. Best wishes on your journey to better health.

Cathy, USA - Fibromyalgia

I was a very busy 40-year-old woman in 1989. I owned and operated a business, used my MA degree to counsel as a volunteer, was active in my community as a board and committee member and was raising a teenage daughter as a single mother.

The last week of a month-long trip to Australia, I came down with what I thought was the flu. I felt no better several months later and I was diagnosed with fibromyalgia at Vanderbilt, confirmed at Mayo Clinic.

The next 20 years were filled with lifestyle changes and trying every medication that came on the market. Some helped the pain and fatigue but the side effects weren't tolerable.

In 2013 a friend sent me the Stanford study on LDN for fibromyalgia syndrome (FMS). I sent it on to my endocrinologist who, with some skepticism, prescribed 4.5 mg at bedtime.

Within 30 days I could see a difference in my pain level. Ten years later I still take 4.5 mg at bedtime. The only side effect I have ever had is increased dreaming which has never been a negative.

I am grateful for those who have worked diligently to bring this medication to the public. It's been a game changer for me.

What is Fibromyalgia (FM)?

There are many overlaps between fibromyalgia symptoms and chronic fatigue syndrome (CFS)/myalgic encephalomyelitis (ME) symptoms but the main difference is stated as pain being the most dominant symptom in fibromyalgia, whereas in ME/CFS fatigue is more dominant. Both conditions are painful and have a serious impact on the quality of life for the patient.

Symptoms of fibromyalgia include musculoskeletal pain, increased sensitivity to pain, chronic sore throat, gastrointestinal issues, post-exertional malaise, fatigue and cognitive impairment.

As with ME/CFS there are no definitive tests that can diagnose either condition. Diagnosis is made by eliminating other known and measurable illnesses and on the presentation of the symptoms. Both conditions can exist alongside one another.

Treatments include various pharmaceuticals such as anticonvulsants, anti-inflammatory medications, antidepressants, sleep aids and psychotherapy (usually CBT). Diet and exercise may also help.

HYPERMOBILE EHLERS-DANLOS SYNDROME

Doug, USA - hEDS

The very next day after my starting dose of LDN was abnormally above average, and so was the next, and the next. I thought it might be working but was cautious. Two weeks later I stepped up my dose and again, the next day set a new benchmark, and it just continued. The week after that I had some crazy long and physically trying days that would have absolutely laid me out. It didn't happen. I was tired but not "down". That's when I knew LDN was really working for me.

A week or two later I stepped up again. I'm currently at the standard dose and I saw increased benefit at each step up. LDN has knocked my daily discomfort down to where it is no longer a top item on my mind; it's there but not usually part of my decision making anymore. LDN is the only "pain" medication I'm on currently. It is completely unlike any other I've tried. Nothing is dulled or blunted and I can still hurt, I just hurt FAR less. I feel like it teaches my body how to feel better. LDN has also reduced my fatigue and required rest and given me incredible energy like I've never had before. I think I'm getting a glimpse at what normal people feel.

Amanda O'Sullivan, BSc, MSc, PhD, PGDip, Ireland - hEDS

As a doctor in genetics with a degree in biochemistry I knew that there had to be a better approach to managing the chronic pain and reduced quality of life associated with the hypermobile Ehlers-Danlos syndrome, which I was diagnosed with. Maximal pain medication and nerve blockers were rendering me unable to function for myself or my family.

I contacted the LDN Research Trust to learn more about LDN, approached my GP and finally found a consultant in Ireland to manage my treatment. I started at 1.5 mg LDN, working slowly up to 3.5 mg so far with a target dose of 4.5 mg. The benefits so far are widespread. I notice significant reduction in nerve pain, increased energy levels, reduced fatigue and anxiety with a significant elimination of brain fog. Bone pain is still present but I can function for more hours in the day after only 30 days on LDN.

This can only continue or improve. I am delighted that I have found a medication that biochemically and pharmacologically makes sense to treat the physical symptoms of my condition whilst allowing me to engage in day-to-day tasks.

The potential of this drug for a myriad of conditions could, in my opinion, change patient mental health and pain management for chronic pain conditions.

What is Hypermobile Ehlers-Danlos Syndrome (hEDS)?

hEDS is thought to be an inheritable condition that affects connective tissue that causes joint hypermobility, joint instability and chronic pain. Other symptoms can be mild skin hyperextensibility, abnormal scarring, chronic fatigue, gastrointestinal problems, dysautonomia and mast cell activation diseases.

The cause of hEDS has not been definitely identified and there is no test available to diagnose it as the gene(s) in which the mutation occurs remains unknown. The diagnostic criteria are general joint hypermobility, unusual stretch marks that have no explanation, recurrent abdominal hernias and other signs of connective tissue abnormality. Family history is also taken into account. Exclusion of other similar conditions is also made.

There is no specific treatment for hEDS but symptom management is usually handled by a range of healthcare professionals – such as physiotherapist, occupational therapist, CBT and genetic counselling which can help you understand the possible cause of your condition. Rarely the faulty gene(s) that causes this condition is not inherited and can occur in a person for the first time. This then can be carried forward to future generations. The patient is also given suitable pain relief and pharmaceuticals tailored to symptoms.

LYME DISEASE

Tore, Norway – Lyme Disease

I take LDN against Lyme disease. Like many that struggle with Lyme I have my diagnosis from a private German doctor, not the National Healthcare Service. Despite long and thorough medical examination, my disabling neurological and rheumatic symptoms remained undiagnosed by the Norwegian Healthcare.

I had no medical history prior to 2016.07.23. On that evening, around eight o'clock, I suddenly felt sick in a very strange way; lightheaded and tired, with high pulse. During the six months to come symptoms increased in number and strength. From an active, healthy, happy, 49-year-old who could run a half marathon, I became a disabled, sad man that spent my days in a chair.

In the end I could hardly walk for five minutes without walking sticks. Social contact, even on the phone, drained me, and I could definitely not work. Dizziness and brain fog were the main symptoms, but I also lost muscle power, most notably in legs and arms. My head ached, ears were ringing, eyes hurt so I could not read or watch TV. I had muscle cramps, shots of pain that came and went across my body, and even the smallest muscles and joints were sore.

I was sent from doctor to doctor, examined from top to toe, but despite my sorry appearance I became one of the invisibly sick. Blood tests were normal except for high levels of ferritin, which can indicate an infection. I received one month of doxycycline pills, that immediately made me feel better, but far from cured me. Despite negative borrelia tests I started to suspect a Lyme infection. I had spent a lot of time outdoors, running and bicycling in the woods. An insect bite from the day I got ill, became a wound that did not heal for several months.

To make a long story short, in March 2017 I went to Germany to see a well regarded specialist on this disease. He diagnosed me and started treatment for Lyme. The next two and a half years I took different types of antibiotics, both pills and IV, up to 2000 mg a day. Antibiotics reduced symptoms, but did not make me completely well.

Based on new American research, my German doctor started treatment with Antabuse/disulfiram. It was more effective and with less side effects than antibiotics. But it did not cure me. After about two and a half years I developed neuropathy, a common side effect of Antabuse, and had to quit. I did not want to go back to antibiotics, so I was pretty sure that there were no options left for me. But in the Antabuse group on social media I had seen that one member used a medication called LDN for support. Maybe it could help me?

In Norway LDN is a controversial medication among many doctors, unless you suffer from MS. I managed to persuade a relative who is a doctor for a prescription. Today I have a doctor that is up to date with LDN and prescribes it to me regularly.

In June 2021 I started out with a quarter of a pill, about 0.75 mg. After a few weeks and some research, I decided to try what is called alternative regime, which I understood to be more efficient against infections. I took 3 mg morning and evening. I have gradually decreased my dose when I have felt the effect lessen. I take a pause one day a month. Today my dose is 2x2 mg.

The only side effect I have experienced is that I do not sleep as well as I used to. And I dream more. I use melatonin to improve sleep, and it helps.

LDN had effect from day one. 0.75 mg immediately reduced brain fog and dizziness, that had returned after I quit Antabuse. But it was when I started the alternative regime that things really started to happen. The effect has been amazing! LDN is not a miracle drug that cured me over night, but gradually over a period of about two years it has improved my health to a degree I never dared to hope for.

Neurological symptoms like dizziness and brain fog, are gone. Ok, on a bad day I can sense them, but they are not inhibiting my life. The same goes for all the other symptoms that I have struggled with for years, loss of muscle power, the painful eyes, aches in joints and muscles. Blood tests show normal ferritin level.

Today I can run more than ten kilometres! I run five kilometres in 28 minutes. That is ok for a man at 55 years. Especially one that was disabled a few years ago. I can also be social, and I am looking for a job!

In addition to LDN I take a blood pressure medication (8 mg candesartan).

I often say that taking LDN has saved my life, but that is only half the truth. It has given me back a life that is very similar to the life I had before I got sick, seven years ago. I am not completely recovered, but I am not sick anymore. I have a bad day now and then. And I still make progress, two years after I started taking LDN. Thank you for the work you are doing!

Annalisa, USA – Lyme Disease

My name is Annalisa. I am 54 years old and live in Sparks, NV USA. I was diagnosed with Lyme disease in 2011. The process to get diagnosed took several months, but I finally ended up with a Lyme specialist who has treated me ever since 2011.

I consider myself extremely fortunate to have had an excellent doctor who has helped me regain my health. After many years of antibiotics and supplements, I was able to get my life back to about 80% of normal. I could function, work again, take care of myself and my family. However, I still had some lingering symptoms such as brain fog, muscle weakness, joint pain, and dizziness that would still flare up. I would treat these flare-ups with antibiotics and herbals and other supplements to get the flare to settle down. This worked for many years, but I still wasn't operating at 100% of my former self.

In September 2019 I had a sudden onset headache in my right temple. This headache was extremely acute and was the worst pain I had ever experienced. This headache was unlike any I had ever experienced before. I took my usual migraine medication and over the counter medications, but nothing would take away the pain. I ended up seeing a neurologist and other doctors about my temple pain, but no one could give me anything that helped. I had every blood test, scan, and test done to check for anything that might be causing the pain. Every test and scan came back negative. The doctors prescribed me pain pills and migraine medications. There wasn't anything that took the excruciating pain away. I was miserable 24/7.

In the summer of 2020, I told my Lyme specialist about my temple pain. I told him how I had seen several doctors and had many tests run and no one could give me any type of medication that would help it. He recommended that I start taking LDN to see if I could get some relief.

I was very excited to start this medication after reading success stories about it. So, in the summer of 2020, I started on 1.5 mg, taking a tablet. The relief was almost immediate. I started to have less temple pain within the first week. I felt like a miracle had taken place!

I stayed on 1.5 mg for three weeks and went up by 0.75 mg every three weeks until I got to 4.5 mg. The pain in my temple finally totally disappeared and I was honestly a new person who was so happy to have my life back! LDN is the only medication that has helped my temple pain and helped me regain my life.

The other amazing thing that has happened to me while on LDN is my lingering Lyme symptoms have been put into remission. After three weeks of being on LDN I noticed that my Lyme symptoms and flares were not nearly as frequent or severe.

Since the summer of 2020, LDN has been the one medication that has helped me regain my life. I tell anyone and everyone how thankful I am that I was prescribed LDN by my Lyme specialist. It is a true miracle and I am so thankful I have my life back and am functioning at 100% of normal! Thank you to everyone who has a hand in LDN!

Lisa, USA – Lyme Disease

I was diagnosed with chronic Lyme disease over ten years ago. My life was extremely difficult with pain affecting every aspect. I was given antibiotics, which were great in the beginning but the long-term effects were difficult to deal with. I took countless medications that had little effect. Hydration therapy and LDN have been what has helped the most.

Dr. Molly prescribed LDN for me ten years ago and the approach taken changed my life for the better.

I had no side effects at all when I started LDN. The only medications I take now are allergy medications, migraine medication and LDN daily. I still have hydration therapy as needed, perhaps once a month.

LDN decreased the severity of my Lyme disease flare-ups, Dr. Molly's innovative approach to chronic illness gave me my life back.

What is Lyme Disease?

Lyme disease is a bacterial infection caught from tick bites. It is also known as Lyme borreliosis. It is easier to treat if caught early though it isn't always diagnosed early enough. The signs are usually a circular rash around the tick bite that resembles a bull's eye though it's estimated that one in three people don't develop the rash.

Diagnosis is difficult due to the symptoms not being consistent and often mimicking other conditions.

The symptoms are muscle and joint pain, chills and fever, neck stiffness and fatigue. Complications of Lyme disease include arthritis, carditis, ocular issues, skin problems and neurological deficits.

Treatment will be given by infectious disease experts, dermatologists and neurologists as symptoms require. Antibiotic treatment is given of varying lengths of time though some patients will find that symptoms of pain, fatigue and cognitive deficits will continue for some time afterwards.

Untreated Lyme disease can progress to serious, even fatal, health conditions such as cardiac arrythmia and inflammation of the brain and spine.

NEUROPATHY

Vicky, UK - Peripheral Neuropathy

I've had peripheral neuropathy for 20 years, which means my hands and feet have a burning sensation, pins and needles and numbness. Neurologists were unable to find the cause and all of the medications they prescribed had terrible side effects and didn't ease my symptoms.

I heard about LDN on a peripheral neuropathy forum and decided to try it. It was very easy to get a prescription and I've now been taking it for two months. I started on 1.5 mg and was told to increase it by 0.5 every week. By the second week of taking the medication, the burning sensation in my feet had stopped.

I could not live without this medication now. Currently I take 2.5 mg, as this is the dose which I feel is the most effective. For my condition, having a diet which is sugar-free and low carb also helps. I just wish the doctors had given me this information many years ago, along with a prescription of LDN. It would have saved me 20 years of pain.

Fay, USA - Charcot-Marie-Tooth Disease (CMT)

I began having neurological issues in my feet as a teen - I found it exceedingly hard to stand for very long. Through my 20s and 30s, my feet gradually became more and more numb, from the toes upwards, and my arches heightened. I sought medical help all from reputable medical institutions, including the Mayo Clinic, but other than an unhelpful diagnosis of "severe sensorimotor polyneuropathy" I got nothing helpful. The only treatment offered was gabapentin/Lyrica, which did little to help and made me excessively dizzy.

A naturopath started me on LDN 4.5 mg. I had few side effects, perhaps a little wakefulness, as I ramped up gradually to the full dose. I have now taken it for about 12 years and credit it with dramatically slowing my decline, with what has eventually been diagnosed as the progressive neuromuscular disease CMT type 2, genetic mutation unknown.

Early on, I was afraid that I could end up in a wheelchair within a decade or two. Little is known about my diagnosed disease - particularly prognosis. With the help of LDN (which I now take at 9 mg per recent research) and PEA (palmitoylethanolamide) - which helps tremendously with neuropathic pain, I am able to function pretty well and can mostly continue to live my life.

Yes, I do have some limitations, but it far less dramatic than I think it would have been without the LDN. My biggest struggle is finding compounding pharmacies who will not price gouge patients for LDN. When you are living on SSDI, even $40-$60 per month is a big chunk of my budget, and neither Medicare nor Medicaid helps cover the cost of compounded meds.

What is Neuropathy?

Neuropathy is disease or dysfunction of one or more peripheral nerves. The symptoms are numbness, tingling and/or stabbing and shooting pain in the affected area, loss of balance and co-ordination and muscle weakness, often in the feet.

There are several types of neuropathy: diabetic neuropathy, Guillain-Barré syndrome, carpel tunnel syndrome, meralgia paresthetica and complex regional pain syndrome.

There is also acquired peripheral neuropathy which can come from physical injury, vascular and blood problems that decrease oxygen thus causing nerve damage, systemic autoimmune diseases, hormonal imbalances, kidney and liver damage which leads to toxic build up causing nerve damage, nutritional imbalances (lack of B12 or excess vitamin B6 being the most common). Several pharmaceutical medications are also known to cause neuropathy.

There are infections that can attack nerve tissues causing neuropathic pain such as the varicella-zoster virus (chicken pox and shingles), and any virus that damages the central and peripheral nervous systems will cause pain. Genetic mutations, either inherited or "de novo," meaning they are completely new to the individual and not present in either parent, can lead to neuropathy.

Correcting underlying causes can result in the neuropathy resolving on its own as the nerves recover or regenerate.

SJÖGREN'S SYNDROME

Brooke, USA - Sjögren's Syndrome

I take LDN for Sjögren's syndrome. I first noticed symptoms start to get bad in August of 2022, but my doctor believes I have had Sjögren's for years. At the young age of 30, I was dealing with extreme fatigue, brain fog/memory issues, numbness in my extremities, dizziness, hair loss, anxiety and depression all relating to Sjögren's. LDN, along with some vitamins, have been life changing.

My fatigue and brain fog have improved a lot and I now only get the numbness on occasion instead of daily. My anxiety/depression is much more manageable as well.

The rheumatologist I first saw was not helpful in treatment. He put me on Plaquenil and I did not see much change in symptoms. I went to a new family doctor and he introduced me to LDN and I'm very thankful.

I started on 1.5 mg of LDN in March 2023 and have increased it every couple of months by 0.5 mg. I am currently on 2.5 mg of LDN and have had no side effects at all so far. I have been taking it for a total of five months. I noticed a difference in symptoms about one month after starting LDN and they have been continuing to improve.

LDN is the only prescription medication that I take along with B complex, vitamin D, vitamin C, and zinc. I'm not 100% yet and this is just the beginning, but I am on the path to feeling normal again. I feel LDN has changed my life for the better.

Iris, USA - Sjögren's Syndrome

I first noticed symptoms in my early 40s. It started with severely dry eyes, fatigue and stiffness. I had to have my tear ducts cauterized. I was given 300 mg of Plaquenil (hydroxychloroquine). I also have thyroid problems and was taking 88 mcg of levothyroxine.

I'd done some research and read a book by Dr. Bernard Bihari and his work with low dose naltrexone. I found LDN to be extremely interesting but had a hard job finding a doctor who would prescribe it. I finally found a rheumatologist who listened to me and he assured me that it wouldn't hurt to try it. I've been taking 1.5 mg of LDN for the last ten months and I'm happy on this dose.

I had no side effects at all and after about six months I realized I had more energy; more movement and the joint pain had practically gone.

I'm still taking 30 mg cevimeline and 200mg of hydroxychloroquine along with the 1.5 mg LDN.

LDN has been the game changer for me. I hope I can continue to take it. I wish more doctors were more receptive to at least try it for their patients. I also wish the insurance would help with the cost because right now it doesn't.

Kristen Schneider, USA - Sjögren's Syndrome

LDN has changed my life! I have Sjögren's and it was debilitating prior to taking LDN. I used to have flare-ups frequently and they could last a week or more. I have been taking LDN for three years now and may have had one or two flare-ups since the LDN started working. It has also helped with brain fog and I don't wake up feeling tired after a good night's sleep anymore. I take 3.5 mg in the morning and 4.5 mg in the evening.

What is Sjögren's Syndrome?

Sjögren's syndrome is a condition that affects the parts of the body that produce fluids, such as tears and spit and other bodily secretions.

The symptoms are dry eyes, mouth, vagina and skin; fatigue, muscle and joint pain, swelling between the jaw and ears (swollen salivary glands) and sometimes rashes, particularly after sun exposure.

Sjögren's is an autoimmune disease that may be linked to genetics or hormones but this is not yet certain.

Treatment includes eye drops to maintain moisture, drugs to increase the production of saliva (pilocarpine and cevimeline), NSAIDS if arthritis symptoms develop, methotrexate and hydroxychloroquine which are classified as DMARDs, being said to treat the underlying disease rather than its symptoms.

MISCELLANEOUS PAIN CONDITIONS

Susi, Canada – Complex Chronic Pain

In 1986 when I was 22, as a back seat passenger, I experienced a traumatic motor vehicle accident of which I have zero memory of to this day. I broke my pelvis, had a traumatic brain injury and fell into a coma for a month. I spent four months in hospital rehabilitating. During that time I was diagnosed with bipolar disorder as a result of my frontal lobe brain injury. I've been taking Lithium ever since. Even with all of that my fractured pelvis has been my Achilles' heel ever since. I feel my entire adult life has been plagued with ongoing and often debilitating chronic pain.

I have done everything! I couldn't accept living in pain for the rest of my life. Besides the obvious chiro, physio, pain meds, I've done cranial sacral therapy, seven years of prolotherapy which helped me the most, until I had a hip labral tear at work. I owned my own TENS machine, etc. I've been to pain clinics. I kept trying for answers.

I know my condition is difficult for doctors to treat, I understand that. Five years ago I spent seven months at a pain clinic where I had hoped to be a candidate for a hip replacement. The MRI, that I paid privately for, showed I didn't need that. There was nothing they could do for me, and I was sent home in tears with an opioid patch that made me sick.

My amazing GP then prescribed Lyrica for me. He explained the trauma to my nerves is why my nerves continuously "misfire." I'm still on Lyrica as I'm bedridden way less when taking it. I saw a new pain specialist last year who took one look at my file, told me I've tried everything and that he was no longer going to inject me. He then suggested I try spinal cord stimulator surgery as a last resort. I became obsessed with learning about it, and we almost flew to the US last September to get the surgery done quickly. The cost would have been $80,000 US which is a lot to us Canadians.

I first heard of LDN through a social media pain group. Everything happened fast. My UK-trained GP agreed to prescribe it for me. I showed him all the LDN Research Trust guidelines and I'm his guinea pig. Dr. O'Brien knew my desperation for pain relief.

I started LDN at 0.5 mg the first week of September and slowly began titration. By November we could see benefits. We went to Disneyland and I had a pain flare the night before which would normally have meant spending the following day in bed, drinking strong alcohol to take the edge off my pain. Instead, I went to Disneyland for 12 hours!! Amazing! In September my big fear was that LDN may not work for me.

While I was increasing my LDN, I was also accepted for the Canadian SCS surgery which is fully covered for me. The Canadian system didn't take as long, and I was able to put the money I saved by not going to Michigan for surgery, into a special savings account for my son who will be going to medical school next year.

I can stay on LDN, get surgery, reduce or eliminate Lyrica and Cymbalta nerve pain meds after surgery. If only I knew 20 years ago about LDN, I could have breathed easier knowing one day there was an answer for pain relief.

LDN hasn't been 100% cure for me but the relief I feel, feels like a miracle. I sleep now. I am thankful to take LDN for the rest of my life, like lithium. Like a diabetic needs insulin, I need LDN. I'm about to fly to New Zealand, something I wouldn't previously have had the confidence to do. I deserve this finally after all the suffering I've had to endure. Thank you to Linda and everyone involved at the LDN Research Trust.

Gemma, UK - Relapsing Polychondritis

I was diagnosed with relapsing polychondritis in 2002. All they could tell me about it was that it was a rare disease with inflammation of cartilage and can affect the joints, ears, nose, throat and lungs – I was figuring all of that out for myself. What they couldn't tell me is what caused it but they thought it was an autoimmune disease. It's a systemic illness and it had caused hearing loss in my left ear, my nose was swollen and my eyes hurt all the time. I felt bad all over. Every joint it seemed was hurting; the pain was terrible.

I was prescribed all the drugs they could think of, one after another; nothing helped. Prednisone, which helped a little, plus methotrexate, cyclosporin, leflunomide, some I can't remember the names of. Then it was a biologic – infliximab I think it was. I had bad side effects to the DMARDs but the biologic wiped me out and put me in the hospital. My throat closed up and I had to have a tube in my throat to keep my airway open. When my lungs became affected, I was told there was nothing left to try and they told me I had maybe six years to live.

I had a friend with rheumatoid arthritis and she was telling me about a drug she'd been taking for quite a while called LDN. She'd found it through a social media RA support group. I didn't listen to her for all those years and I really wish I had. I thought she'd just gone into remission and gave this little-known drug all the credit. I was rather wary of drugs at this point.

Being desperate now, and in so much pain that my life was barely worth living anyway, I asked her more about it. She gave my daughter some internet links and my daughter read about it and said I should try it; how could it hurt?

My daughter came with me to see my rheumatologist; I had run out of steam by now and knew I couldn't argue on my own – and I did expect an argument. At first my rheumatologist dismissed it as snake oil but my daughter had printed off a lot of information and she pushed him, saying that nothing he had done had helped so it would be unfair of him to deny me this chance. We left the information with him and a fortnight later his secretary called to say that he was willing to prescribe LDN for me, as he knew there was nothing else to try. To be quite frank about it I'd lost all hope and without my daughter I would never have been able to put this case forward. I expected maybe six more miserable years. It doesn't only affect the inflicted, it affects the whole family, so I also felt guilty for their suffering having to watch me struggle with the pain and misery.

So it was now 2009 and I finally got my LDN. I started slow on 1 mg, I was a little worried, although my daughter had explained the side effects were minimal, particularly compared to the other drugs I'd been on. Not much happened so I went up to 2 mg, then 3 mg over a period of three weeks. I felt somewhat nauseous for a week or so; my daughter explained it could be like a detox reaction from what she'd read. The nausea passed. I wasn't sleeping well but that wasn't unusual given the pain I'd had. I gradually got to 4.5 mg by about week four and then one morning I woke up and there was no pain. I got out of bed and walked, by myself, to the bathroom. It was a remarkable feeling. My sleep improved, my mental state lifted beyond measure, I had hope!

This was 15 years ago and I now feel "normal". Not as perfect maybe as someone who had never been through this disease but so much better that I can live a relatively normal life. I have felt better for the majority of the time since starting LDN. I still flare occasionally but it isn't totally debilitating and it doesn't last long, maybe a few days. I didn't get my hearing back in my left ear but that's nothing – the pain has gone! When I flare it's usually when I've overdone things; been stupid in other words.

I lost seven years of my life, being in pain and torment. I suffered the side effects of all those drugs, on top of the illness itself; and all the while there was a simple harmless drug called LDN that would have helped me. The damage done to my body needn't have been. How this drug isn't used as a first line treatment is beyond my comprehension. However, I can't live in the past with regrets and I have years of life ahead of me and I am so grateful for LDN. Better late than never, it has truly given me my life back.

TJ, USA - Birdshot Chorioretinopathy (Uveitis)

My name is TJ and I'm now 71 and retired (female). I've always lived in the northwest US. I was diagnosed with birdshot chorioretinopathy in 2015. It is a rare autoimmune (1:250,000) form of uveitis, always bilateral, considered blinding without therapy. The "usual" therapy is some type of immunomodulating drug such as methotrexate and a large but tapering dose of prednisone. I refused the drugs, wanting something better, something that would not impact me systemically.

I started taking LDN within about six months. The visual symptoms abated almost immediately but figuring out a dose was challenging. We experimented a lot with the dose. My symptoms were greatly decreased but my ophthalmologist said I still had worrisome retinal inflammation.

I found a specialist at Kaiser who offered to inject intravitreal ILUVIEN implants, a miniaturized implant with nano release steroid expected to last three years. These were implanted late in 2017. My vision has been amazing, perfect 20/20, no glasses, better than all my age peers.

I stayed on the 4.5 mg LDN all this time. Why, when the implants worked so well? It's been kind of like a security blanket I could not let go of.

At five and a half years now, well past the expected implants' range of effectiveness, my vision is still crisp and all test results are normal. My doctor's clinical exam reveals no signs of inflammation.

My doctor is surprised the implants lasted so long. Is it because the LDN has supported the implant therapy or because my birdshot is progressing very slowly? We will probably never know. I will continue with the LDN 4.5 at bedtime six out of seven days.

Cindy, USA - Mast Cell Disorder/Histamine Intolerance

After losing my gallbladder and 60 lbs several years ago I began to feel fatigued all the time, I had brain fog and an overall feeling of being off. While teaching an art class at a local art center my tongue began to swell to the point of not being able to swallow. I immediately drove myself to the fire/rescue station a few blocks away where they administered an injection and took me to the ER via ambulance. I was there approximately 16 hours during which the swelling happened several more times. I was released with a diagnosis of an unknown allergic reaction and referred to an allergist who informed me that it had not been an allergic reaction but mast cell disorder.

During the following year I worked with a holistic ARNP who further diagnosed me with histamine intolerance. After taking a myriad of supplements and expensive testing I was no better. As a matter of fact I was worse.

The anaphylactic reactions and hives continued sending me to the ER every couple of months. I realized at that point that if I didn't become an advocate for my own health I wasn't going to get any better so I began doing extensive research about both conditions, treatments and possible physicians. I made an appointment with an integrative doctor at Mayo Clinic.

He ran additional testing, referred me to a dietitian and ultimately suggested LDN as a mast cell stabilizer. Through additional research I located an LDN specialist who worked in conjunction with my doctor to begin my treatment at a low dosage titrating up to the recommended 4.5 mg.

I've now been on LDN for approximately one year. During that time I've regained my energy, the brain fog is clearing, the hives are almost gone and I haven't been to the ER in nearly a year. My healing journey continues and LDN will definitely remain an integral part of it.

Angela, Denmark – HIV/AIDS

In early 2003 I was pretty healthy, then by the summer things started going downhill. My hair started falling out and I had chronic back and joint pain. By 2004 I had chronic diarrhea and fatigue so bad I could no longer function. The brain fog was terrible and I was just getting sicker and sicker.

My blood work was awful and I saw so many doctors' numerous times – one telling me to see an oncologist who gave me bone biopsies which were negative. It was only because they could not figure out what was wrong that one doctor finally said he'd give me a HIV test. That came back positive, I was devastated.

I was put on highly active antiretroviral therapy (HAART), which most HIV patients end up on at some point. What was amazing was that after 3 months on this medication, and supplements and herbs, I felt a lot better but the side effects weren't good. I had elevation of liver enzymes, awful rashes and nausea.

I wanted to come off the HAART but they told me that I had to take it for the rest of my life. It was a very toxic drug and would probably have killed me in the end so I came off it anyway. I felt well again, despite the side effects, but didn't want to be on that drug for the rest of my life. I took plenty of vitamins and minerals but got no support from my doctors about the things I was taking or for coming off the HAART.

I researched more and more and eventually came across LDN. I went to my doctor and asked for it – they didn't want to know about it at all.

Two years later I saw an alternative doctor and he agreed to prescribe it, he was quite eager to read my research and to learn for himself.

That was 7 years ago. When I first started taking LDN I felt that it helped me in a short amount of time, I had no side effects at all! I started to feel more energetic, slept a lot better and my head was clear. My AIDS symptoms have been perfectly stable and it's so good not to have the side effects of the standard AIDS medication.

I forget actually that I have anything wrong with me! I don't get colds when other people get colds, I feel fantastic. Thank God that a harmless drug is available to solve immune system problems, all the standard care drugs come at a price to your wellbeing, LDN increases wellbeing while modulating the immune system. Why isn't this tried first?

Sarah, UK – CRPS

LDN has changed the canvas of my life. A diagnosis of CRPS following spinal injury, surgery and lasting nerve damage. A deterioration over the years, bed bound and increasingly isolated from the physical world. I was trying everything. A clinician myself, I had explored all that allopathic medicine could offer. Having used and worked with complimentary therapies and holistic practice for decades, I continued to integrate that into what little quality of life I had. But flare-up followed flare-up and my body began to shut down more and more. Chronic fatigue, cardiac arrhythmias and balance problems evolved.

Purely from my own research, 18 months ago, I discovered LDN. I gradually titrated my dose up to 4.5 mg daily and after about three months I began to feel a little more energy return to my body. It was brief at first and I had to consciously "rein it in", sometimes successfully, sometimes not! Over the next few months, alongside further development of my spiritual practices, a little more energy returned. Maybe only enough to cook a meal, which probably isn't much to most people, but to me it was huge.

Gradually that evolved to short walks, albeit with a stick, but without being wiped out for weeks. Managing my pain continued to be a daily journey and flare-ups were ever present but they didn't crush me for weeks on end. My dysfunctional immune response, that is a fundamental part of CRPS, also seemed to be improving.

Nowadays I am able to enjoy walks with my dog and I can feel myself getting stronger. Any progress feels painfully slow and I have had to radically adjust my expectations but I have hope again. Hope that I can live a life with some fulfilment. Hope that I can heal and prove those consultants wrong who had written me off. Hope that I can enjoy quality time with my children. LDN has given me stability and strengthened my resolve to keep moving mountains.

Patty, USA – Histamine Intolerance

I was diagnosed with histamine intolerance by a functional medicine doctor in August, 2020. My second functional medicine doctor also stated I have long COVID in October 2022.

I was prescribed lorazepam 1 mg 3 x day for the histamine intolerance which helped until I took a few drops of grapefruit seed extract that intensified the lorazepam and now I'm tolerant to lorazepam.

My first functional medicine doctor mentioned LDN but I didn't pursue it. Then my biological dentist recommended LDN because I couldn't get my reactions stable. In early February 2023 I decided to try it after seeing it mentioned frequently on the MCAS social media page. I went to see my PCP who didn't know about it but she knew I'd done my research and she graciously agreed to prescribe.

I started at 0.25 mg and increased to 1 mg twice daily, 12 hours apart, which is what I'm using now. I use the compounded transdermal cream.

The side effects that I had, that were possibly due to LDN, were lack of appetite, as food doesn't taste normal, more muscle aches, though I'm not sure it was the LDN.

I started realizing benefits at the five day mark. Better sleep, I was no longer waking with panic attacks, I had reduced burning in my limbs, better breathing, overall more energy but still fatigued. My inflammation is much less so consequently I have reduced swelling and muscle pain and burning. In hindsight I wish I had started LDN sooner.

CANCER

Anna Murphy, MPharm, Ireland – Pancreatic Cancer

I never once imagined that I would hear the words "pancreatic mass" and "liver lesions" echoed regarding my mum, Virginia, who was just 61 years young. Virginia was admitted to hospital via accident and emergency for worsening symptoms that only a few weeks prior, the GP's receptionist had advised her to purchase an antacid instead of fixing her an appointment.

Amid pandemic restrictions, I was offered a special permission to enter the hospital to sit with Virginia for 20 minutes or so after they broke the devastating news to her when she was on her own. The doctors knew what it was, I knew what it was, but we had to tick the boxes and play the waiting game, and nothing will haunt me more than the sad glaring look in the medic's eyes; for treatment to commence, a biopsy had to be carried out along with further scans and tests.

A week or two into February 2021 and we had it in black and white, "adenocarcinoma on the head of the pancreas with multiple metastasis to the liver." As a qualified pharmacist I knew what this meant, the prognosis was that my mum only had a few months left to live.

Up until the official diagnosis and indeed until my mother's final weeks, I had researched obsessively. Pancreatic cancer is one of those neglected cancers in terms of funding, research and available treatments. Despite the fact that one in four people with pancreatic cancer die within a month of diagnosis, mainstream research still has not found a cure, except if the cancer is caught early enough for surgery. It is also one of those cancers that comes with a whole multitude of complications, some very predictable, causing very fast declines and can halt the commencement or continuation of treatment.

As a pharmacist I'm well aware how conventional medicine has improved and extended the lives of many all around the world, and so there is a need for pharmaceuticals, however, conventional medicine has failed people with pancreatic cancer miserably. The available chemotherapeutic options supposedly extend life, but the evidence suggests that this is only fractional and the question remains, at what cost? Some patients are lucky where they can maintain a decent quality of life while on chemo for pancreatic cancer but for many the suffering due to chemo side effects can be too much. The only other options are experimental, with clinical trials being suggested to Virginia by her oncologist.

I also carried out informal searches, joined online groups of cancer patients and carers and there were very few positive stories of people recovering with conventional treatment only.

In my literature search I had come across a case report by Berkson, Burton M et al. "Revisiting the ALA/N (alpha-lipoic acid/low-dose naltrexone) protocol for people with metastatic and nonmetastatic pancreatic cancer: a report of 3 new cases," 2009. The authors discuss their patients who were diagnosed with advanced pancreatic cancer with metastasis and who had achieved remission on a protocol called LDN/ALA. Finally, I found something that was promising as clinical presentation of these patients mentioned in these reports were very similar to my mother's clinical presentation. I dug deeper, educated myself on LDN and ALA and other integrative/alternative protocols such as high dose IV vitamin C and their role in oncology. I gathered the published scientific evidence, printed it out, and presented it to the registrar who was our face-to-face HCP looking after Virginia's case at the oncology clinic.

The registrar had never heard of LDN as a treatment option. I asked him to prescribe LDN which is an inexpensive, low-risk, efficacious treatment that at the very least can be beneficial for inflammatory symptoms and at the most can help terminal cancer patients achieve remission; but despite his ability to legally use his clinical discretion he told me he couldn't prescribe this. The fight for my mother's life had just become frustratingly even more difficult than it had to be; just another barrier.

I continued my search and had come across a private clinic in Glasgow, Scotland, and had initiated the process of requesting LDN from the clinic – that also took time as there are few such clinics in the UK and there was a high demand with a long waiting list for an appointment. While we waited for our private virtual appointment, Virginia had further declined and then her routine appointment at the NHS oncology clinic in Belfast had come about.

At that NHS oncology appointment, Virginia finally got a face-to-face appointment with her oncologist, he who didn't even look at the evidence that I attempted to show him for LDN and immediately dismissed any possibility that it could work. Even as an HCP myself, to this day I still cannot comprehend why our overstretched, financially strained healthcare system promotes certain experimental treatment options for patients (clinical trials) when there are safe inexpensive alternative and potentially lifesaving treatments available with some evidence supporting their efficacy.

Evidence comes in many forms, and while I completely agree that the most robust evidence is found in randomized controlled trials (RCTs), requiring a lot of financial input, I also believe that we (HCPs) should not by default immediately dismiss other forms of evidence without looking at it - this sadly seems to happen within the NHS. For LDN the likelihood that there will ever be a fully comprehensive RCT is low, as this medicine is now off-patent, meaning it is no longer a financially attractive venture for investors. Therefore, for repurposed medicines, including LDN, we must be open to consider other evidence forms i.e., support the collection of real-world data and use the available data in our clinical decision making process. I believe it is our duty as carers within the health industry to widen our scope and consider other options such as repurposed medication*/alternative therapies; especially in cases like my mother's when the patient is faced with only two conventional options; one of which offers nothing but a few extra weeks of life (a couple of months at most) and the other being an experimental treatment with an unknown benefit-risk profile.

Through the insight that we gained as a family caring for my terminally-ill mother together with my knowledge as a pharmacist, I find it unsettling that HCPs are not utilizing their skills, professional judgment and clinical discretion to offer a patient a potentially useful and safe alternative, particularly in cases like Virginia's when it is so very clear that the treatment algorithms based on RCTs and designed by authorities offer little to nothing to the patient.

When researching I learned that LDN is useful in multiple therapeutic areas and there is a plethora of evidence, coming from individual physicians and patients globally, from different clinics and private practices. Some of this evidence is published in black and white in the medical literature, like that of Berkson et al. mentioned above. The available evidence points to an improved quality of life and even remission for patients suffering from very serious illness. The question for me will always remain, why would anyone deny a person who has been classed as a "terminally ill" patient the chance to try this repurposed medication with an already long-established benefit-risk profile? There are very few unknowns about this off-patent medication, after all, naltrexone was first approved in 1984 and there is a global lifetime experience of its use in clinical practice. In these supposedly hopeless cases such as Virginia's, where conventional medicine offers little to nothing to the patient, is the plethora of available real-world experience on LDN not evidence enough to support the prescription of LDN?

As LDN is not an option in our mainstream healthcare system, there was a delay to discovering it. This delay, along with the barriers placed in front of us by our NHS, directly impacted my mother's cancer journey and potentially her overall survival of the disease.

When Virginia was finally established on LDN therapy, the benefits she saw in herself, and that we saw in her, were remarkable; except for times when she was an in-patient and the last ten days or so of her life. Virginia slept better, experienced less pain and had no requirement for heavy painkillers such as morphine that are often prescribed easily in patients with pancreatic cancer in their last months and weeks. Anyone who has ever cared for a loved one with "terminal" cancer and who are dealing with complications of pancreatic cancer, will have felt a huge weight being lifted when they see improvements in their loved one's quality of life.

However, when Virginia experienced complications associated with her disease, and she was hospitalized, her integrative/alternative medicines were confiscated on admission each time. She was not supported to continue her private treatment as an NHS inpatient.

While I cannot state with certainty, I firmly believe that, from the moment Virginia was diagnosed, had we been offered access to and the chance to establish, and the support to maintain the ALA/LDN protocol, then she would have had an entirely different and less distressing cancer journey and may even still be with us. However, without the education of NHS HCPs, support for them to prescribe and hence support to their patients, how will we ever know the full benefits that this medication could have had on patients like Virginia? Perhaps, Virginia could have fully benefited from LDN and maybe even survived, but now we will never know!

Virginia, passed away in the local hospital on 21 June 2021, just three weeks past her 62nd birthday leaving behind her husband, brother, five children, five grandchildren and a sixth grandchild "baby Rice" who is now on the way.

In loving memory of Virginia Murphy nee Cahill (29 May 1959 – 21 June 2021)

* Drug repurposing (DR) (also known as drug repositioning) is a process of identifying new therapeutic use(s) for old/existing/available drugs. It is an effective strategy in discovering or developing drug molecules with new pharmacological/therapeutic indications.

Micha, Canada – Blood Cancer

I take LDN for migraine, pruritis, fatigue, bone and joint pain related to my blood cancer (polycythemia vera). My symptoms started almost 20 years ago with migraines and fatigue. It was hard to work as the migraines were becoming increasingly debilitating and my former employer was getting upset about the amount of sick time I was taking. I took sumatriptan for the migraine for years but, as effective as it is for treating migraines, it did not prevent them and it does nothing for my other symptoms.

LDN was first suggested to me by my naturopath, but she couldn't prescribe it. I have a great GP who is willing to entertain many hairbrained ideas that I bring to him, so I'm lucky. I showed him a study I found online showing that LDN helps migraines and he was happy to give it a try. Since seeing my success he says he has started to learn more about LDN and try other patients on it!

I started LDN in October 2022, initially on 1 mg a day. Dosing is still a work in progress. I found 2 mg/day helpful for migraine etc., and at the advice of my naturopath I have tweaked this a bit. I am on LDN for the anti-pain effects, but on the off chance that it might improve my underlying disease state (the blood cancer). I am doing a modified dosing schedule that is a hybrid of standard cancer and pain dosing. LDN for cancer is ideally done in "pulses" and not daily. So, I currently do a bit of a wackadoodle dosing schedule of Monday- 3 mg, Tuesday – 3 mg, Wednesday – 1 mg, Thursday – none, Friday – 1 mg, Saturday - 3 mg, Sunday - 3mg. I noticed more insomnia since first starting, when I took LDN at night, but I take marijuana oil to offset this, and I find it's no longer a problem when I switched to morning dosing.

It started to work slowly. In the first month I noticed a mild reduction in migraine days. After three to four months I noticed a big difference. Unfortunately my pharmacy messed up my prescription renewal at one point and so I went two weeks without LDN and my migraines came back in full force. This showed to me just how effective the LDN is. It took another month after this trip-up to get me back on track and now I feel like every month I'm just feeling better and better.

I only took two other medications before LDN, sumatriptan and apixaban (an anticoagulant), and I still take those now, along with the LDN, but I rarely need the sumatriptan any more.

LDN means I can continue to function as a productive member of society and as a mother. It has given me my life back. Unfortunately my blood cancer (polycythemia vera) is incurable and so it's something

I must live with for the rest of my life, however with LDN I feel like I can continue to function much better.

Before starting on LDN I thought I may have to quit my job and go on disability as I was having so many migraines that I couldn't reasonably work. I had to take a year off of my master's degree as well. A year ago I thought I was on a slow downward spiral towards disability and ultimately, death. LDN has given me my life back! I can't say enough positive things about it.

Since starting LDN I have only had to take two days off work due to pain, and I am back working on my master's degree. I am able to show up as the kind of mom I want to be (energetic, engaged etc.). It does not feel like an exaggeration to say it has saved my life! In addition to this it has improved my bloodwork, so I have a hunch it might also be helping the underlying disease process and not simply my symptoms.

I think LDN should be a standard part of the pharmacological approach to myeloproliferative neoplasms, as it treats so many aspects of these diseases; pain, fatigue, pruritus, all have been improved by LDN. I thank my lucky stars I was fortunate enough to be introduced to this miracle drug!

I really hope LDN is studied in the context of polycythemia vera and other chronic blood cancers as it's been a godsend for me!

Michelle, UK – Breast Cancer

It was January 2018 when I first noticed a lump in my breast. I did nothing about it for a month because, well basically I didn't want to think about it, it couldn't be THAT! But it was whirring away at the back of my mind, this thing that only happened to other women, not me. Eventually of course I went to the doctors and was examined and I was told that it was basically a blocked milk duct, duct ectasia she called it. I was advised to use warm compresses and it would likely go away on its own.

Feeling much relieved I went home and used warm compresses until I started forgetting about it. Six months later I noticed that it was swelling and there was redness and the lump itself seemed a lot bigger than before. Thinking it had possibly got infected somehow, I didn't worry but I went back to the doctor, figuring I'd get antibiotics.

The doctor referred me immediately to the breast clinic and I had a biopsy that day. Now I was really worried and not just a little bit annoyed that the doctor had "assumed" something without tests and had therefore misdiagnosed me. I was told it was quite a rare form of breast cancer called inflammatory breast cancer – quite an aggressive cancer that affects the lymph vessels in the skin of the breast, they are invasive ductal carcinomas developing from cells that line the milk ducts of the breast and then spread to the skin. So, I had stage 3 breast cancer, the good news being, the doctor said, that it hadn't spread outside of the breast but would require a lot of chemo and radiotherapy.

I didn't really have time to process the situation, my husband didn't seem to be taking it in properly either. However, it all got very real when I was immediately booked in for 7 rounds of chemotherapy. Then a mastectomy, followed by lots of radiation. It was a horrible time for me and my family. I was told, at the end of treatment, that I was extremely lucky to be in the top 10% of people who respond to this treatment regimen, there were hardly any cancer cells at all on subsequent check-ups. Yes, I was lucky but I didn't feel lucky, I'd never been so ill with the surgery, chemo and radiation – it took a lot of getting over.

Consequently, when I found a lump in my neck, just above my collar bone, two years later, I was devastated. Having had cancer previously, this time I was immediately sent to oncology for tests. It transpired that I had a cluster of four small tumours in my neck, above my collar bone. Back to chemotherapy for 6 months. During this period, I was reading all I could find on alternative cancer treatments. I bought lots of supplements, changed my diet and exercised when I could rake up the energy. At my 6-month checkup I had a scan and it showed that the tumours had increased in size. It seemed hopeless at this point.

They wanted me to have more chemo, different chemo – more drugs, but I'd had enough so I refused. I carried on with my diet and supplements and research and found many testimonials about low dose naltrexone. I printed all the information I could find on LDN and took it to my doctor; she did her own research on it and obviously knew that I'd refused further standard cancer treatment. Within a few days I got a call to say that she was happy to prescribe LDN for me. I was excited because I really felt that this would help – I now believe more in the personal stories of others, who have had results, than all the studies on the internet. At least people's stories are real.

I got the LDN in June 2022, a month after the last scan that had shown growth in the tumours. Then in the November I had another scan and the tumours had shrunk by half. Another benefit, that I wasn't expecting, for some reason, was better sleep, more positive outlook on life, and less aches and pains in my hips and knees (something that had been a bit of a nuisance for a couple of years).

I didn't have side effects with LDN, perhaps a week of vivid dreams but they weren't bothersome. I'm more positive about things now, which will also help the whole situation on its own! I still stick to the anti-inflammatory diet that I started, I still take many supplements – basically anything that eases inflammation; like curcumin, liquorice, ginger, green tea and Essiac tea – those sorts of things, and I feel great! The cancer is still there but it was shrinking at the last scan and I believe it will show on the next scan, which will be in July 2023, that it will have shrunk more. I am feeling very positive. I can't feel the lump in my neck now and it isn't affecting me at all.

I strongly believe that LDN is the game changer for this cancer, the supplements and the diet help of course, but things really shifted once I'd started LDN.

Mayuko, Japan – Tumour Pain
I have been on LDN since mid-January 2023 and currently at 3.0 mg. I've had no issues with side effects and the pain in the tumor site which had given me a hard time to lie down/sleep has gone away. I wished I had started earlier and not let fear get in the way!

Claire, UK – Brain Tumour
I have been using LDN (3 mg once a day) since 2015. LDN was prescribed by my consultant Professor Angus Dalgleish at St. George's

Hospital in London. Prior to this I had my tumor debulked (which removed 80%). I then had the standard NHS treatment of radiotherapy and chemotherapy. I had three different types of chemo. None of them made any difference to my tumor. I was even put on palliative care.

I was then introduced to Professor Dalgleish who suggested I try LDN. The last MRI scan I had showed that my tumor has disappeared - neither Professor Dalgleish or I could believe it. I continue to take LDN now, have an MRI once a year and I am back driving too.

LDN and Cancer

Naltrexone (NTX) is an opioid antagonist that inhibits cell proliferation in vivo when administered in low doses. Naltrexone in low doses can reduce tumor growth by interfering with cell signalling as well as by modifying the immune system. It acts as an opioid growth factor receptor (OGFr) antagonist and the OGF-OGFr axis is an inhibitory biological pathway present in human cancer cells and tissues, being a target for the treatment with low dose naltrexone (LDN).

Clinical trials have proposed a unique mechanism(s) allowing LDN to affect tumors. LDN shows promising results for people with primary cancer of the bladder, breast, liver, lung, lymph nodes, colon and rectum. This short review provides further evidence to support the role of LDN as an anticancer agent.

Ricardo David Couto and Bruno Jose Dumêt Fernandes, "Low Doses Naltrexone: The Potential Benefit Effects for its Use in Patients with Cancer", Current Drug Research Reviews, 2021;13(2):86-89.

LONG COVID

Kayla, USA – Long COVID and Hashimoto's

I've been taking LDN for long COVID and Hashimoto's. I first started having long COVID symptoms in July 2022, and I started taking LDN March 2023. Nobody knows how to treat long COVID yet so I tried a variety of over-the-counter treatments but nothing was helping the long COVID symptoms.

It wasn't difficult to get a prescription for LDN because my doctor puts all of his long COVID patients on it. I started at 0.1 mg and I'm currently at 0.75 mg. I'm still titrating my way up to find my best dose. I had side effects the first two weeks, and sometimes when titrating up. The side effects were headaches, dizziness, insomnia, and vivid dreams.

I noticed improvements the very first day even with the side effects, and I have continued to have improvements with each month and each increase in dosage. I currently take about ten medications, but LDN is definitely in my top three most helpful that I can't be without. It has helped me go from basically bed-bound, to functioning much better than before.

Alicia, USA – Long COVID

I take LDN for long COVID which I developed after I contracted the delta variant and was vaccinated in May of 2021. I became bedridden. I was experiencing tachycardia, histamine intolerance, anxiety, depression, brain fog, debilitating fatigue, confusion, internal vibrations, and unsteady vision. I couldn't work or watch my small children for long periods of time and I felt myself falling into a depression. I had trouble finding the strength in my arms to wash my hair in the shower and would often use a chair to take breaks from household chores.

Doctors prescribed SNRIs, hyperbaric oxygen, ozone, and massive amounts of supplements, none of which made any noticeable difference in my abilities to live life. Fortunately, my ND knew about LDN and thought it could help me. I started LDN in the beginning of 2022 at 0.5 mg and am currently at 4 mg which seems to suit me. The only side effects were vivid dreams, which I still sometimes have, but they are much less bothersome than they were when I started.

I remember in the beginning of taking LDN I told my ND I didn't think LDN was doing anything for me. She saw my abilities slowly increasing and life coming back into my being and encouraged me to keep with it. Within four to five months I started being able to go back to work for longer and longer periods of time. I was then able to do things like attend my son's soccer games and actually go to the grocery store more often than Instacart orders.

I believe that LDN is still making improvements in my life to this day. I continue to improve slowly and sometimes find myself feeling 100% again which I didn't think was possible. It's truly allowing my body to heal. I am not on any other medications.

Taking LDN means that I get to be a part of the life that I once took for granted. My kids get to look for me and smile as we make eye contact as I sit in the audience at sporting events or school functions. I am actively living without repercussions of "overdoing it" and my kids get their mom back

Camille, USA – Long COVID

I had COVID starting in November 2021 and then it kind of peaked around the last week in November. Then in the months that followed I had some long COVID symptoms, some of which resolved on their own and some of them didn't.

When I had COVID it messed up my liver enzymes. Something was off with my liver and my thyroid, and while my liver issues resolved, I was having some gallbladder pain, but I couldn't get a diagnosis despite definitely having some gallbladder pain.

I also was having some prolonged shortness of breath. There were a lot of episodes of rapid heart rate, especially when I would first stand up. I would get out of breath really, really easily and was just really fatigued all of the time. The exhaustion comes with COVID, but for me it wasn't resolving. So, those were the main things that were really persisting.

My experiences when first taking LDN was subtle. I started with one pill for a week, and then I slowly moved up to four pills. I think I was at 5 milligrams, a really low amount. Once I was at that higher dose the changes I noticed were that my heart rate over time totally normalized. I didn't have that exhaustion anymore. I actually have had more energy than I had since I have started having kids. Huge change there. I didn't have the achiness in my body.

I had pretty severe adrenal fatigue onset right before COVID started, and then COVID obviously made it worse. I noticed all of my symptoms from that had resolved after starting LDN and that was an additional bonus. The energy change was huge, and the gallbladder pain completely resolved almost immediately after getting up to that full dose.

As far as side effects go, I have crazy dreams since starting LDN, which I actually like. Getting to sleep is really easy now and the dreams are super fun. There were no negative side effects whatsoever.

I really appreciate that my doctor took the time to educate herself on something that isn't really fully out there, and a lot of people don't know about. I'm just grateful that I have LDN.

GASTROINTESTINAL

Harry, USA – Ulcerative Colitis

I suffered from ulcerative colitis for about ten years starting in 2001. None of the then-current medications were able to solve my problem and the only solution, as stated by my doctors, was to remove my colon.

Upon doing a number of years of research on IBD I found that a number of patients with numerous conditions, including IBD, were finding relief with the use of low dose naltrexone (LDN). This drug, off patent for decades, is normally used in the treatment of drug addiction; it is an opiate antagonist, at the dose of 50 mg per day. As defined, "low dose" is anywhere from 1 mg to 4.5 mg per day. Every physician I have discussed this with agrees that at this low dose it could not possibly do any harm and yet, with a very few exceptions, the physicians refused to prescribe the drug.

Due to my condition, ulcerative colitis, I was unable to acquire outside health insurance and am dependent on the VA for my healthcare. Every physician at my center in San Antonio claims that:

"They cannot write outside prescriptions" – this is not true, I have a copy of the VA memo that says otherwise

"They can't prescribe 'off-label'" – this is not true, doctors do it all the time

"A physician could lose his license if he prescribes 'off-label'" - also untrue.

"No research has been done on this use of LDN" – this is not true;

I have furnished them with information of studies including those of Dr. Jill Smith of the Pennsylvania State University College of Medicine that was first published over a decade ago.

Let's talk about me and my experience with LDN and my ulcerative colitis.

In late 2011 I finally found a physician who would not only discuss LDN, he prescribed it at a dose of 4 mg per day. The drug companies that make this drug only make 50 mg tablets for the use stated above for drug addiction. That being the case the smaller doses have to be made up at compounding pharmacies. In addition to the LDN, I added green smoothies and rejuvelac (This is a raw food made by soaking a grain or pseudocereal (usually sprouted) in water for about two days at room temperature and then reserving the liquid). I also removed all gluten and dairy from my diet. I also stopped the 5400 mg a day of the Lialda (mesalamine) that had proven to be ineffective for years (from the VA that cost them over $1500.00 per month). I asked my doctor about also dropping the 150 mg per day of Imuran (another $600 per month for the VA) and he said to keep taking it. It has some very nasty side effects including possible cancer.

Since starting LDN and adding all of the above changes to my diet the results were just short of miraculous.

I saw a change in my IBD symptoms within a week and after having been on LDN and new diet for about five and a half months I had a colonoscopy in late February and the results said "appeared normal." Additionally, all biopsy results were clear with only "signs of inactive ulcerative colitis."

I might add that now I've been taking LDN for over 12 years; no ill effects and I eat anything I want. The gluten free and "no dairy" regime went away and in that entire time I have had NO flares and numerous scopes - all negative.

And yet, even with these results, the VA physicians still refused to prescribe LDN. They finally agreed, after the February 2012 scope, to taper off the Imuran which I did.

So, the bottom line is that the VA, and most of the "mainstream" physicians, in my opinion "those that are afraid of something," I'm not sure what, would rather give a patient a couple thousand dollars a month of drugs that don't work, cause the patient to suffer in numerous ways and then declare the fix is to remove the colon which, unless someone knows something I don't, is irreversible.

My VA doctor stated to me that his source for "Nobody knows anything about this" is "the drug companies." The drug companies can't make any money on a drug that has been off patent for years so it's not in their best interests to "know" about the efficacy of something as cheap and harmless as low dose naltrexone.

The cost of the compounded LDN was, at that time, about $15.00 a month and, for me at least, it works.

I am aware that it may not work for everyone, but at the very least it seems to me that it might be good to try it before taking the drastic step of surgery.

The cost really is not an issue for me. However, how many other patients are being left in the dark about alternative treatments in lieu of major surgery? Additionally, how much money is the VA wasting for drugs that do not work?

Something is very wrong with our system and it would seem that nobody cares. Whatever happened to "do no harm?" Removing someone's colon without trying a change in diet and a drug "that couldn't possibly hurt at this dose" seems callous and irresponsible.

Laura Fisher, MD, USA – Microscopic Colitis

I am not positive about where and when I learned about naltrexone, but I think it was in a book I read about ten years ago called Google LDN! by a Mr. Joseph Wouk about his successful use of naltrexone in treating his multiple sclerosis.

With no pre-existing gut disease whatsoever I learned I have microscopic colitis by getting a biopsy from my colon at a screening colonoscopy. Then I learned there was no effective treatment; I tried it all. I was 62 years old and had had no previous serious illnesses other than strep throat at age 4, treated with injectable penicillin.

I changed my diet dramatically by eliminating all grain foods, sugar and several foods identified as diarrhea-provoking from a stool examination for IgG. My current diet includes fish, shellfish, vegetables, fruit and nuts (some call this pesco-vegan.) I also found some definite relief from using Pepto-Bismol tablets as per publications by Kenneth Fine, MD. Once I began taking 4 mg of LDN nightly along with the Pepto-Bismol (8 tablets daily), I stopped experiencing diarrhea.

I tried 1 mg of LDN at first and worked up to 4.5 mg which seemed to give me a slight hangover so I reduced the dose to 4 mg. I experienced zero adverse effects on 4 mg.

I did find that I require both the Pepto-Bismol AND the LDN to give me the relief I needed.

Mainstream medicine offers a cortical corticosteroid as treatment for MC, but it only works in about one third of patients and tends to stop working on them after about a year.

Chantelle, UK – Crohn's Disease

I started having very mild symptoms that slowly got worse and I was told it was IBS. I was offered anti-spasmodic drugs. Gradually the symptoms got worse until eventually I was vomiting quite regularly, in constant pain and only eating small amounts of food.

I had a colonoscopy and I was told I had Crohn's disease. They put me straight on to prednisone, I was only on that for 3 or 4 weeks before I started feeling puffy, my skin felt squishy as though I was full of water. I wasn't a fan of the weight gain, I didn't need more weight. So, I came off that and they gave me methotrexate – that lasted a month, so four doses, before I couldn't tolerate the side effects of that any more. It just seemed to make everything worse and I was so fatigued on that. Then another immune suppressant – mercaptopurine, which I was told would reduce the need for steroids, but I was pretty determined to avoid steroids after the last experience anyway. Mercaptopurine seemed to deal with the Crohn's symptoms somewhat but took a long time to work, I felt no benefit for about 4 months but the side effects were a good bit quicker. Did I want to swap my Crohn's symptoms for bad skin, hair loss and oral lesions? Why can't they develop drugs that don't mess people up in other ways?

I got sick of experimenting with different drugs that just made me feel worse in different ways and I started researching what I could do for myself for Crohn's. Diets and supplements were heavily featured so I changed my diet and bought some supplements but, although feeling better for trying, I had no real faith that that's all it would take.

Then I happened to come across low dose naltrexone (LDN) on a support group for people with gastrointestinal issues. I looked on other sites and read academic papers, that stated "We don't fully understand the mechanism of action but it does seem to do something ..", pretty much like many other drugs, they rarely seem to know why something works, and clearly don't know what else it might do that's not so beneficial.

I was extremely sceptical because there are so many claims for LDN, for so many different diseases, that it sounded like a bit of a joke really. One drug, small dose, practically no side effects, making so much positive difference to so many people with so many different illnesses? So, I dismissed it.

I'd stopped taking the mercaptopurine after about 6 months because I was feeling miserable with the side effects and I thought, maybe with the diet and supplements, that coming off it I'd maybe not be as bad as before anyway. Wrong. I felt terrible, I started feeling nauseous again and could barely eat.

I started thinking about LDN again, there must be something to it right? I printed off the information and took it to my GP, fully expecting him to dismiss it, like I had. And he did. So I went back to the LDN Research Trust website and found a prescriber on there. It was so straightforward I was kicking myself for not doing it months before.

By the end of the second week of starting LDN my symptoms had gone. Just like that. And the only "side effect" that I had was actually positive – I felt happier, less stressed, less tired. If that's a side effect bring it on!

A month after being on LDN I went back to my GP, just to tell him how good I felt. He saw an obvious change in me that did pique his interest and now he's actually looking into it. I feel he doesn't want it to be LDN that's made such a difference so quickly, but spontaneous remission isn't it, that's not what happened at all.

There are some academic papers showing, and proving, that LDN is helpful in Crohn's and IBD – they conclude that LDN has a direct effect on intestinal epithelial wound healing, this has been proven with scans and endoscopes. I had converted my doctor and I'm thrilled because now other people will also benefit. He can not deny the scan images in the academic papers online, they speak for themselves.

I'm so glad I found LDN, my only other options would have given me a miserable life due to side effects of drugs, even if the Crohn's symptoms had remained in check. And the best part is that LDN regulates the immune response, whereas standard treatments suppress the immune system making patients more likely to suffer infections. What's not to like about it?

Edythe, USA - Intestinal Adhesions/Blockages/Inflammation

My symptoms began 2016 culminating in a blockage in November 2019 and laparotomy to untwist my intestines. Daily life was debilitating. I was unable to eat for fear of another blockage - no elimination for a week to ten days. The bloat and pain was continuous. Once elimination was achieved then I had 12 to 16 hours of constant all-over unrelenting abdominal pain.

The pain affected my daily life and outdoor activities and sleep. I was homebound for two years. The only treatment was pain medication offered by gastro doctors and PC. I did not like the mind-altering effects of opioids so used only heating pad and sustained myself with organic Kate Farms feeding tube nutritional drinks.

I came across LDN on YouTube and researched it. I spoke to my primary care doctor about LDN and he wrote a prescription for a compounding pharmacy. I began at an ultra-low dose 0.01 mg and every two weeks increased until 0.05 mg. All pain subsided within six weeks and I raised the dose to 1 mg.

I now experience NO PAIN; it is heaven living without pain. I gradually began eating soft foods and soups. The only side effects were temporary anxiety and startle response and vivid dreams. These all subsided as time passed.

I now enjoy full sleep and a calmness; I no longer stress about when and if pain bouts will come as they do not. It has changed my life remarkably and I am a proponent of LDN for reducing inflammation within my body.

Debbie, USA – Ulcerative Colitis

I take LDN for ulcerative colitis. I started on 3 mg about 16 years ago. It took me about a year to increase to 4.5 mg because of muscle spasms that I already had, but the increase seemed to make the spasms worse, although the blood and mucus symptoms stopped, but I have irritable bowel as well.

I've been in remission for approximately 15 years except for a couple of flares. Over the years I have managed to increase to 4.5 mg. I have celiac and LDN seems to cause my reaction to gluten to be delayed by about six hours.

When on 3 mg my energy level, muscle and joint pain were greatly improved but 3 mg did not help UC. On 4.5 mg the pain is better than before LDN but not as reduced as it was on 3 mg. I will take LDN as long as I'm alive.

Jean, UK – Crohn's Disease

I started LDN for the management of Crohn's disease in 2018. I was diagnosed on 27th of September 2015. They still have not been able to tell me the type of Crohn's disease. The symptoms were mild but they found ulcers in the intestines. I did not want to go onto the conventional medication after seeing what it did to my husband who has arthritis. I managed somewhat with the specific carbohydrate diet and then found the LDN website.

I searched for a chemist within the UK and found one in Glasgow. I had my consultation and was prescribed sublingual LDN. I started on one drop and worked up to nine drops per day. No side effects apart from wonderful sleep. The Crohn's disease is under full control with normal bowel movements and no pain. I have passed my incredible results on to others in order to spread the word. Thank you, thank you, thank you.

John B. Monaco, MD, USA – Ulcerative Colitis

I have been using LDN, personally, for nine years and prescribing it for more than ten years. I was diagnosed with ulcerative colitis and for 25 years, I could not resolve the underlying inflammation in my colon. I was able to control the symptoms with a functional medical approach. My conventional colleagues could only offer expensive biologics with significant side effects or surgery.

After starting LDN, the inflammation had resolved within a year and has, to this day, not returned. I have had similar success with my patients for a variety of conditions from autoimmune thyroid and sarcoidosis to inflammatory bowel disease, celiac disease, eczema and psoriasis. I call LDN the wonder drug of the 21st century. With few side effects, LDN has made a difference in so many lives.

Donna, UK – Crohn's Disease

I first had symptoms about 10 years ago, very mild and not too concerning, but uncomfortable now and then. Around 4 years ago things started getting unmanageable; I had cramps in my stomach, bloody loose stools and a fatigue that seemed to creep up on me and wouldn't go away. I hadn't had a great appetite for a while but that got worse, I didn't really want to eat and I was thin enough, I didn't want to lose more weight.

I had a really bad flare one night and it was really shocking, I was so ill and ended up at the hospital. Then it was back and forth to the hospital for a few months until I was prescribed some drugs that would help somewhat. I was pretty miserable with side effects from then on and still had some symptoms of Crohn's, not as bad but the side effects just replaced any mild improvement.

I do read a lot so I'd researched diets and found the specific carbohydrate diet which did help some but it didn't make me as well as I wanted to be. I wasn't happy about being on the steroids and immune suppression drugs that the gastroenterologist had given me, I didn't know whether I was better or worse really.

More reading, and several Crohn's support groups later, I heard about LDN. Feeling sceptical, I read people's experiences of LDN and wondered whether it could possibly work for me. I was doubtful because I'd had these symptoms for a long time. Searching "LDN and Crohn's" specifically I came across a study written by Leonard Weinstock called "Efficacy of Low Dose Naltrexone in Patients with Crohn's, Colitis and Ileitis" and I was really excited that there was a drug that could help me that didn't seem to have the horrible side effects that I was suffering with the immune suppressants and steroids.

I'm happy to say that for the last 9 months, since starting LDN, I've been more than fine, I've been great! Not just my stomach either, I feel generally mentally better too. I'm just normal now, as good as I could be. I still eat the same, I got used to the diet and quite enjoy it and occasionally I'll eat forbidden foods without issue, like chocolate, but I find I'm not really too interested in sweet things. I no longer take any of the drugs given to me by the gastroenterologist and haven't missed them at all, or the side effects.

If I'd had LDN at least 4 years ago I would have had that many more happy years but it wasn't to be. I have LDN now and for that I'm really grateful. But without my research, and my unwillingness to accept that those awful drugs I was given were the only option, I don't know where I'd be. Miserable I guess, or asleep for the main part as the immune suppressants caused so much fatigue, or worse – going for surgery to remove lengths of my intestines!

I'm glad I searched and found LDN, it has made all the difference to my quality of life. For anybody wondering about whether to try it or not I would say just try it, there's no harm in trying it at all, and it might just change your life.

LDN and Gastrointestinal Inflammation

Around 30% of patients with inflammatory bowel disease (IBD) are refractory to current IBD drugs or relapse over time. Novel treatments are called for, and low dose naltrexone (LDN) may provide a safe, easily accessible alternative treatment option for these patients. We investigated the potential of LDN to induce clinical response in therapy-refractory IBD patients, and investigated its direct effects on epithelial barrier function.

Conclusions:

Naltrexone directly improves epithelial barrier function by improving wound healing and reducing mucosal ER stress levels. Low dose naltrexone treatment is effective and safe, and could be considered for the treatment of therapy refractory IBD patients.

Lie, M. R. K. L., et al. (2018). Low dose Naltrexone for induction of remission in inflammatory bowel disease patients. Journal of translational medicine, 16(1), 55.

MENTAL HEALTH

Lisa Mainier, DO, PhD, USA

I first learned about low dose naltrexone, LDN, when I attended a lecture on how to treat long-haul COVID and COVID vaccine injuries. The lecture focused on the upcoming viral season, how to treat those suffering long-term side effects after COVID infections and those with post COVID-19 vaccine syndrome. I was surprised to learn how the use of low dose naltrexone works overall to decrease inflammation. I learned that LDN modulates the immune response by promoting the function of T-Cells and NK-Cells and also decreases the release of proinflammatory cytokines such as Il-6, Il-12 and TNF. By regulating lymphocyte response and reducing mast cell activity, the robust immune response caused by viral proteins and other pro-inflammatory proteins can be held at bay or regulated in such a way that the immune system does its job protecting the body, without over-reaction and destruction to the body. After taking courses offered at the LDN Research Trust, I also learned of the benefits of LDN for mental and emotional disorders such as PTSD, for which there are few completely satisfactory treatments and for which there are so many associated emotional and health issues.

I just started introducing low dose naltrexone in my practice as a part of a holistic treatment option for complex PTSD, in addition to outside psychological counseling and coaching. My first patient was diagnosed with complex PTSD due to negative childhood experiences in the family and then later in the medical setting during COVID. He "stepped up" psychological counseling and added professional coaching in an effort to respond to events in a more meaningful way. He realized he lacked tools to help him navigate the complexities and ever-changing circumstances in his social, professional and personal life. He had tried medications in the past, all of which caused intolerable side effects, personality changes, sleep issues; and carried a stigma in the medical setting which did not allow the most appropriate care for other medical conditions. He had tried EMDR, a special therapy for PTSD, which helped a little, but he reported no lasting effects. "I could not see the end of treatment. What would that look like." He continued counselling, a cognitive behavior therapy approach in addition to personal coaching. He felt there were benefits but needed more to stop the intrusive thoughts that re-hashed the recent trauma he had witnessed in the hospital during COVID.

After discussing how LDN may work for this patient and offering literature and citations for personal research, the patient voiced an interest in starting LDN. It was discussed and agreed that the patient would need to continue counseling and therapy as part of the process. It was explained that during the dose adjustment period, there may be times of worsening thoughts and symptoms, as the brain may become more aware of another perspective of influences. He may become aware of thoughts from which he was protecting himself.

The dose was started at 1 mg of LDN for two weeks, at which time there were no changes. He had noticed some minor GI and dream disturbances after the first dose. After beginning LDN 1.5 mg for two weeks, there were no changes and after ten days he wanted to increase to 2 mg of LDN. There were few GI and sleep side effects, however he reported having transient periods of sadness and anger for a few days "out of nowhere." After ten days, he began the 2.5 mg dose, which he quickly increased to 3 mg for ten days without much change, still noticing a few days of transient, unprovoked anger and irritability. In fact, during this time, he reported having a conversation with his psychotherapist about what thoughts were based on actual present events as opposed to past events. He reported now being able to determine the difference between a reaction to past events and worries about events that are not occurring in the present. He was able to determine that in the present, he is safe, despite what his body was trying to tell him. Once he was able to tolerate the 4 mg dose without GI side effects or sleep issues, he noticed retrospectively, that he really was more present in the "now" and spending less time "stuck" reviewing past events that had been so emotional.

Upon further discussion, he was able to articulate that he can live in the present without reviewing the past traumatic experiences. He explains that he can think of past experiences of abuse and recent traumatic events, if called upon to do so, but no longer feels the same emotional rush of anger, frustration and sadness. He reports feeling much less vigilant. The thoughts do not provoke the same emotions that they had in the past and he hadn't really noticed it until his partner happened to mention less stress in the home. "There is no more walking on eggshells in the home. I am no longer falling into a rage about the slightest of triggers." He explains that even though there are situations that are not perfect, he sees them from a different angle, a challenge to determine how to deal with life issues that were once so upsetting. He reports feeling less weight on his shoulders. He no longer has to "wait" for disturbing images of the past to play in his mind. He claims he does not experience the same anticipation of fear, frustration and anger from past "stories", which is so freeing. He explains that "life did not become perfect, but my view is less fearful."

This patient did not get to 4.5 mg of LDN, which was the goal. He is happy to be taking 4 mg of LDN every night. He sleeps well and denies any GI effects. He denies vivid dreams. He does not report feeling as if the effects of LDN wear off over the day, but remarks when he skipped LDN for a few nights before bedtime, he noticed a little less tolerance for annoyances through the day. Upon realizing he had not taken the LDN for a few nights, he took the 4 mg dose in the daytime and noticed no untoward effects. He now takes 4 mg LDN every night. He is taking no other medications at this time, as anti-depressants and anti-anxiety medications "did not work for me at all."

At this point, he reports a healthy respect for things that may go wrong in life. He expresses, "There are disturbed people who could damage a part of a person's life and there are bad things that could happen, but mostly, there are good people in front of us every day that support the idea of compassion for others. Bad things may happen, and maybe they are lessons to be learned. If my mind is clear and I have the tools, perhaps I can work my way through the bad and see the good for what it is. LDN has helped me see things clearly. I may still have memories and emotions, but they no longer run my life."

Low dose naltrexone worked for this patient, my first patient. My goal and hope for the use of LDN for this patient was to simply enhance his psychotherapy. I underestimated LDN's effects. As per the patient's own report, he did not realize that he had let go of some emotions that seemed to be ongoing reactions to the past trauma that did not belong in the present or with situations that were unrelated to past events.

This was my first choice because this patient was not on any other medications. He wanted to change, to stop reacting to spontaneous visions of the past. The visions and their associated reactions were significantly reduced.

I will continue to offer this option to other patients dealing with trauma and other emotional concerns. Now, however, I would like to begin with patients afflicted with multiple autoimmune conditions for which they are left effectively untreated, those with chronic allergies, energy concerns and other symptoms for which there is no concrete diagnosis or treatment for which LDN has been studied or witnessed to be beneficial.

The use of LDN in my practice is just one more option for those who seek answers to conditions for which they have been told are "all in your head," because "you are just old" or are due to "nervousness and anxiety." Those are just not acceptable explanations to symptoms for which there are no easily explained and understood etiologies or specific medications available. In my practice, if the answer is not obvious, it is time to dig deeper and investigate fully!

Jeff Barris, PharmD, USA

I have asked psychiatrists who have non-responding patients to try an LDN protocol appropriate for that patient. After a few months of discussion, John walked into the pharmacy with symptoms of depression, sleep issues and problems with memory, focus and concentration.

With the MD's authorization, I placed John on LDN 0.5 mg and slowly titrated him to 2.5 mg at bedtime. John walked into the pharmacy today, after two months of LDN therapy, and with tears in his eyes, to let me know that he has his life back. He feels great, sleeps great and can think clearly. John had not felt this way in over 20 years. It was quite gratifying and heart-warming to hear this outcome.

In turn, LDN and myself won the trust of my local practitioners and this allows us to make a difference.

Nat Jones, RPh, FAPC, USA

I first heard about LDN around 2009 when I started getting prescriptions for multiple sclerosis from neurologists for us to compound. The list of diseases for which it was being prescribed gradually increased over time.

Dosages at that time were primarily 1.5 mg, 3 mg and 4.5 mg immediate release capsules, with 4.5 mg being the highest dose prescribed. Occasionally we got requests for transdermal applications in pediatric autistic patients that weren't able to swallow capsules.

In the beginning approximately 70% of the MS patients got regular refills, but I wasn't tracking any data then. From that I deduced that it must be beneficial otherwise they wouldn't continue to spend the money.

I have one particular PTSD patient that has had a dramatic turnaround in their functionality with 1 mg twice daily of LDN. He served two tours in the US Air Force in Afghanistan which left him with debilitating depression to the point of not being able to hold a job. The drug therapy offered by the Veterans Affairs practitioner was ineffective and caused bad adverse effects leading to discontinuation.

After being on LDN for just two weeks in 2019, he could tell a difference in his mood which led to progression in other areas such as exercise and lifestyle. He states that he never wants to stop taking this for fear of relapsing and calls LDN "lifesaving."

Judy Tsafrir, MD, USA

I am a holistic psychiatrist. Patients consult me because they are suffering from symptoms related to brain health. The health of the brain is related to the degree of inflammation in the body. The degree of inflammation in the body is related to a person's immune status. LDN helps with inflammation by modulating the immune system.

It is rare that I do not suggest a trial of LDN to a patient, because almost everyone could potentially benefit as most psychiatric conditions are mediated brain inflammation.

When a patient has an autoimmune condition that is accompanied by psychiatric symptoms, they are even more likely to respond. It sometimes can work wonders in conditions for which conventional medicine does not have much to offer; those conditions that are mysterious and poorly understood like chronic fatigue syndrome or fibromyalgia.

Because LDN is safe, inexpensive and sometimes a game changer, in my experience, it is worth trying in almost every case. It does not help everyone, but it almost always makes sense to initiate a trial, as the potential benefit far outweighs the risk.

NEUROLOGICAL CONDITIONS

Linda Elsegood, UK - Multiple Sclerosis

My life was perfect but hectic. I had two children. I ran the home and did all the cooking, cleaning, gardening, and decorating; I was the taxi, studied, and worked full-time. I was Wonder Woman! I thought I could do anything and everything. This was 24 years ago, in 2000.

I was happy and healthy, which I took for granted. One day, I came home from work, and my father phoned to say that my mother, who I was very close to, had had a severe heart attack. I rushed to the hospital, and I sat beside her bed for 48 hours. I thought if I went to sleep, she would go to sleep, and that would be it. In hindsight, it was ridiculous but made sense to me at that time. When my mother came out of hospital, she had to have somebody look after her, and my father was in a wheelchair. So, I had my parents stay with me, and I had to return to work. A very close friend was a nurse; she came to stay and helped look after my parents. The stress and trauma had a massive effect on me. I was so unbelievably tired I felt burnt out. I had no energy to do anything, and strange things were happening. I wanted to go away and have a vacation to feel okay when I returned. I just needed to get away from all the pressure and stress.

My husband could not take a holiday because of work commitments, so I took my youngest daughter. We went to Portugal for a week at Easter time, it should have been hot but it was freezing cold and raining; we could either stay in or walk in the rain. We chose to go out in the rain, the rain was hitting us in the face, my left-hand side of my face went numb as if I'd had a filling; I put it down to the rain. (Crazy or what!) Then, the left-hand side of my tongue felt as though I'd eaten something really hot, and it had burnt it. I tried to act as if everything was normal for my daughter.

When I got home, I went to my doctor, who made an appointment for me to see a neurologist.

While waiting four months to see the neurologist, many different things happened. I caught the flu, had gastroenteritis, and a tooth abscess. I got double vision and lost my hearing in my left ear. The fatigue was unbearable; I dragged myself out of bed, drove to work, came home and crawled into bed. I couldn't cope with working five days a week, so I reduced my hours to four days a week, but that didn't make any difference. At this point, I "crashed" and was too ill to work, and became bedbound, I could barely move or stand and used a wheelchair.

The neurologist examined me and said he thought I had had a mild stroke or a foreign disease of some kind, a brain tumour or multiple sclerosis. He doubted it MS because it didn't cause hearing loss. I didn't really like any of those options. I would have liked something that could be fixed with a pill or something. I had an MRI, lumbar puncture, multiple blood tests, and evoked potential tests for my eyes and ears; after all the tests, I was told it was MS. This was August 2000.

I had a three-day course of intravenous steroids. Six weeks later, I was given another course of intravenous steroids because they thought I was going to lose my hearing and my eyesight completely. Oh boy, was I scared! The steroids made me put on so much weight. I'm pale, and my face was like a red beach ball. It was unbelievable. I didn't look like myself. The second course of steroids didn't work. At that time, I was so ill I was on the toilet the whole time. I didn't have any bladder or bowel control. My bowels, I know it's not the done thing to talk about one's bowels but to explain, it was like sneezing. You know how you feel a sneeze coming, and you go achoo? It was like that from my bowels - there was no control at all. I didn't want to leave the house. It happened every day, but never at the same time, which would have been more convenient.

I had no balance; I had to furniture walk. People with MS will know what I mean by furniture walking. I would trip and stumble over nothing. I had terrible vertigo, so if I turned my head too quickly, everything would spin. And my legs became as though they were rubber bands; I used to bounce a lot. I ended up on the floor most of the time for no reason. The numbness on my face and my tongue spread. And after a few weeks, you could draw a line right down my face, half of my nose, tongue, cheek, and chest. I lost the strength on my left side, which was numb with pins and needles, but numb in a way that any clothing or bedding that I touched was really, really painful. I had twitching muscles, restless legs and burning limbs. Like I had sunburn. And they used to be on fire. And I used to say to my husband, feel my legs - they're on fire. He would touch my legs and say, "What are you talking about? Your legs are cold?" To me, they were on fire.

Cognitively, oh my goodness, English became my second language. I couldn't recall vocabulary. Everything was foggy. I would say, "Could you make me a cup of tea?? I never ever drink tea. My husband would say, "Don't you mean coffee?" And I'd say, "Didn't I say coffee?" "No". I would say, "Why do you keep correcting me if you know what I mean? You're depressing me. I think I'm saying it correctly". He would reply, "I'm telling you so you'll know for next time". It doesn't work like that because I think I'm saying it correctly. It was so tiring to try to put a sentence together, which, to me, made sense, but to other people, I was talking nonsense. It made me not want to speak.

The fatigue was so bad that it was exhausting to try to put a sentence together. Often, I would fall asleep while talking or while someone was talking to me.

I needed help drinking as I couldn't find my mouth; I would choke on food. Everything was such a struggle; I sounded as if I had a stroke. I had to speak slowly to try and make sense of my thoughts.

The only saving grace was I slept most of the time. I was asleep about 20 hours a day. I was only awake for 4 hours, which was a blessing as I felt nothing while sleeping. I had intense pains in my head, about 3" in diameter, which would move from the front to the back of my head.

I was prescribed powerful painkillers, which only took the edge off. It was a trade-off as the painkillers made me so nauseous, I couldn't move as I thought I would vomit. I had optic neuritis, where I felt as though somebody had stuck a pencil in my eye to move my eyeball up, down, left or right - really, really painful.

Sometimes, just sometimes, when waking up, I would feel "normal" for 30 seconds before I felt all the symptoms return. I used to pray that one day, they wouldn't come back.

I only left the house for the hospital, doctors or dentist; I had no social life.

Moving forward to October 2003, I saw my neurologist, who examined me. He sat down, looked at me, leaned across the desk, held his hand out, shook hands with me and said, "I'm really sorry to tell you you're secondary progressive now". He got up, opened the door, and said, "There's nothing more we can do for you". And showed me out. I was stunned there was no plan B! Once in the car, I said to my husband, "he may as well have said, go home and die quietly. Don't make a fuss; you're an embarrassment." I felt totally alone and frightened because I couldn't live my life feeling as helpless and hopeless as I did.

One day, my doctor came to visit and brought more painkillers. I was in the house alone. He fetched me a glass of water, and I asked him if he thought I would get any better; he said he thought if I was going to, I would have done by now.

My parents were so upset seeing me like this, saying if they could take the MS from me, they would, as they had had their lives and I was still young (47 years old at that time). I hated seeing the look in everybody's eyes, family and friends. They felt helpless, wanting to help, and there was nothing anyone could do. I had the tablets and thought that my family would understand if I took them all. I wanted to give everyone their lives back; I was stopping everyone from living the life I wanted them to have. I thought they could carry on with life once they overcame the shock. (I now realise this wouldn't have been the case) I felt like a failure; the days passed without me participating, and I couldn't do anything. I couldn't achieve anything. I then thought, who would find me? It would have been my 15-year-old daughter, and I couldn't do that to her. So the only option was to fight it, to do something so that I could actually live again. There had to be something I could do; I had to prove the neurologist was wrong.

With considerable effort, between many toilet visits, I sat at the computer; I could only do 10 minutes at a time, then take a 3 to 4-hour nap. I thought I couldn't be unique and that there must be other people like me; I wanted to know what they were doing. Finally, I heard about low-dose naltrexone (LDN) and people taking it, and everybody said the same thing: if LDN didn't work for me, it at least wasn't going to do any harm.

I found Dr Bob Lawrence in Wales, who sent me a printout to take to my doctor to see if they would prescribe it. I went to see my new doctor, who was very kind and understanding, and she said she would give the information to the partners and I was to return in two weeks. I went back, and she said she couldn't prescribe it for me, but if she were in my position, she would like to try it herself. If I could find somebody who would prescribe it for me, she would be happy to monitor me.

Dr Bob Lawrence prescribed it for me; I started taking LDN on 3rd December 2003, and just three weeks later, the brain fog started to lift; I could think again, which was such a big deal. I wasn't talking rubbish anymore. It was the start of getting my life back.

My 15-year-old daughter Laura spent the whole of the summer holiday doing an excellent job of looking after me, washing me, feeding me, and washing my hair. It was a role reversal. And guess what? She's now a nurse! I gradually got my balance back. Now, when you consider the years of me not being able to carry anything because of the furniture walking and the falling over, carrying a glass with anything in it would've just been too dangerous. One day, she asked me, could you get me a glass of orange juice? And I thought it had been a while since I'd fallen over.

I think I can do this. So, it was all in slow motion - going to the cupboard, getting the glass out, putting it down, opening the fridge, pouring the orange juice in, taking it to her. I didn't fill it right up in case I spilt it, but I took it to her, and I came back and said to my husband, "I've just taken Laura a glass of orange juice, and I didn't spill it!" To me, that was the first really, really big thing that I'd done in a very long time. I'd achieved something; it was such a big deal. I don't think she realised how cognitively impaired I was; I thought I was suffering from some form of Alzheimer's. I thought everything would go; my memory was the only thing I had left. And that was slipping away from me. And that was my biggest fear that I would lose myself completely. Laura came in with the empty glass, put it on the countertop, and said, "It was very kind of you to bring me a glass, Mum, but you didn't put any orange in it". Because of my state of mind, I believed her and not myself; I thought I had imagined putting that orange in there, and I just burst into tears, thinking, well, that's it, I have lost it. Laura said, "No, no, no. I was joking!" I had totally believed her and not myself.

After only 2 months, I came to a crossroads: what did I want to do with my life? Did I want to carry on as best as possible, or did I want to help those people in that deep, dark place I was in? There was no contest; I wanted to help other people who, like me, have been told nothing more can be done for them. LDN is worth trying. It isn't a miracle drug; it's not a cure, it doesn't necessarily help everybody, but it's worth investigating.

It took five months to set up the charity, and now the LDN Research Trust has been established for 20 years. This is a significant milestone. And we've helped over 100,000 people around the world get LDN. It can work for any condition with an autoimmune component, pain, mental health, etc. So far, there are 174 conditions that people have tried LDN for with some level of success, many like mine, that are life-changing.

When you tell people that LDN can be used for all these different conditions, it loses some credibility because it sounds like it's too good to be true. It sounds like a panacea. And anything that's considered a panacea has veracity problems.

Now, for myself, the numbness and pins and needles went, the vertigo went, the balance problems went. I had my bowel and bladder control back. Cognitive things cleared. My eyesight is not as good as it was, but it's okay. The hearing in my left ear is back to 75% of what it used to be, but it is still okay. And it's incredible. I can achieve things. I know I've got MS. I'm not back to how I used to be, but if I plan things and pace myself, I can do anything, which is amazing! I have a life again! Unfortunately, I still get sick and catch things, and symptoms return, but once I get over whatever, they settle down again.

I set up the charity so that nobody would ever get paid. I work without financial pay; my payment is when people I've helped get LDN, who have found it very difficult to obtain, and when they've been on it for a while. They come back and say, "Thank you so much", "I feel like me again"" or "I feel I've been given a second chance", or "I feel I've been given my life back". That is just intoxicating. It's absolutely amazing. Suppose my suffering was to have any meaning. In that case, I've used that suffering to help my fellow human beings by reducing their unnecessary suffering in this particular and very expansive manner. It's been worth it to me.

The most common questions I get are: does it need to be prescribed by a medical physician? Yes, It does. Is there a listing of physicians that people can access, whether it's in the UK, the United States, Canada, or Europe? Is there a list of physicians willing to work with people with LDN? Yes, but they can be hard to find. We now have a list of medical professionals who work with patients and LDN in many countries. Suppose anybody is interested and would like to find a doctor or pharmacy in their area. In that case, the list is available on our website under "find a prescriber" or "find a pharmacy".

The risk-benefit factor is very favourable. LDN handles the inflammatory portion of many conditions really well for most people, which is beautiful. It has certainly been a beautiful thing for me.

Karen, UK – Multiple Sclerosis

I had suffered symptoms for a couple of years before getting a diagnosis of MS in 2005. I looked at all the treatment options, checked out all the drugs that were offered, and decided that I just didn't want to risk those side effects on top of what I was already experiencing. I know a lady with MS who did all of that and I watched her continue to decline and suffer additional problems with side effects of the drugs

– I didn't want that.

Instead, I started reading as much as I could and visited many places online where people were sharing their experiences of living with MS and the treatments they were on. Low dose naltrexone was an alternative drug that seemed to be mentioned a lot and with much enthusiasm. I checked out all the side effects and was pleasantly surprised to learn that they were minimal, some people having none whatsoever! Then I went to my doctor and he refused to prescribe LDN – which isn't unusual from my understanding. A lot of people seemed to have trouble with their regular doctors and consultants.

I eventually managed to find out where all these people were getting prescriptions from and located a private doctor who would accommodate my request. I kept my expectations reasonable; I know it doesn't have beneficial effects for everyone but the odds were in my favour as I'd read that 70-80% of people trying this drug had some benefits, some life changing – though I dared not hope for that.

I started on 3 mg and have never altered my dose in 17 years! All this time my MS has been relatively stable with no other intervention. I am no worse now than I was at diagnosis. Perhaps it's because I caught it relatively early on, when the symptoms weren't debilitating? I know I was lucky enough to have an MRI on my brain early on with my symptoms; the vision issues and occasional muscular weakness, some coordination problems – all of which are resolved now. I can get fatigued now and then but a bit of self-care sees that right in no time. I feel I've dodged a particularly nasty bullet with the discovery of LDN and for that I am eternally grateful.

Lucus, US – Parkinson's Disease

I first noticed that my right arm wasn't moving when I walked, I was getting stiff but had put that down to age related things and never really gave it a lot of thought. The arm started to bother me though, I'd started paying attention to it and it became really evident that something was wrong. I went to a doctor and he immediately said, without any tests, that I had Parkinson's. I was shocked by the diagnosis but decided not to start the medication immediately.

I saw another doctor who told me, after lots of tests, that I didn't have Parkinson's! I was elated of course and went home feeling much relieved. Several months later I found that my arm was getting really stiff, difficult to move – I had a sense that it wasn't responding to signals rather than just being stiff from arthritis or whatever. I got an appointment with a neurologist. He said I had Parkinson's. I was devastated.

I spend a lot of time on the internet and I'd looked into Parkinson's treatments and wasn't really looking forward to the possible side effects of those drugs, it seemed that mental issues were the common side effects, memory issues and cognitive deficits – I really didn't want that, not on top of all the worry about the diagnosis.

While searching for natural means of helping Parkinson's I came across low dose naltrexone. First, I looked into the possible side effects of those – I really wanted something natural, not a pharmaceutical, but I was intrigued enough by people's testimonials that I kept on reading.

I found a local pharmacy online that mentioned LDN so I went in to talk to them about it. The pharmacist explained to me that LDN might not take all of my symptoms away, may not even entirely stop the progression, but it would help my immune system which would indirectly help the Parkinson's and also, probably, allow me to use the minimum standard medication given for Parkinson's. He went on to explain how it was an excellent addition to many generally toxic drugs to mitigate any side effects.

I started LDN 7 years ago and had no side effects whatsoever. It did help a little with the arm stiffness but helped a lot overall. I've always been a poor sleeper and with the LDN I dream a little more but I do wake up feeling much more refreshed. I have noticed that I no longer suffer from colds and the common bugs that come around. When other people are ill, I don't get ill, I don't seem to catch anything that's going around.

I can't say that my Parkinson's is much better particularly but I do think LDN slowed the progression. I'm now 14 years since being properly diagnosed with Parkinson's and when I look at other people with Parkinson's, who have been diagnosed for only 4 or 5 years, I'm not as bad as they are, I don't seem to have quite so many of their symptoms or a worsening of the symptoms I do have.

I go to a group once a month and meet up with other sufferers of Parkinson's, it's a kind of support group, I've made some really good friends there, and it's been helpful but I see a lot of them getting worse over time – whereas I don't feel I am, not so quickly anyway. Only one other member of our group and started LDN, as he was intrigued when I was telling him about it, we have yet to see how he fares on it. A few of the others have asked their neurologists about it and have been put off by the responses they got. Of course, the neurologists don't know anything about it but choose to disparage it anyway. That scared them off I guess. Though I feel it's a real shame that they haven't been given the opportunity to try it, just because the neurologist has an opinion on something he knows nothing about.

I would say to anybody who wants to try something that won't harm, and could possibly make all the difference, to at least try it, you might be pleasantly surprised. You will at least have lost very little if it doesn't work for you in some small way. I'm glad I did, I attribute my relatively good health, compared to some, and the slow progression of this horrible disease to LDN.

Katharine, France – Multiple Sclerosis

I was diagnosed with MS in 2014 when I was admitted to hospital with numbness down my right side. This symptom was not problematic but the doctor wanted to be sure that it wasn't a mild stroke. An MRI and lumbar puncture confirmed the diagnosis of MS.

I was offered all the mainstream drugs but chose not to start any course of treatment at the time. I spent several months researching other options and found LDN.

I translated all the relevant information I could find on LDN (as we live in France) and discussed it with my local doctor. He was in agreement that I should not, at this stage, start any of the mainstream drugs but was ok with me trying LDN.

While I was still researching LDN I had an episode of optic neuritis and received a course of IV steroids. After this episode it was clear that this wasn't just a "one off" so I contacted Linda at the LDN Research Trust to ask how I went about getting LDN. After submitting my medical dossier to the prescribing doctor in Glasgow I was prescribed LDN. I started with the liquid on the advised minimum dose of 0.5 mg and worked my way up to 4.5 mg per day in the evening, however I found this dose too high and dropped back to 3 mg. I now take 3 mg capsules every day.

I did struggle with extremely vivid (and tiring) dreams which did not go away after the first few months, so the doctor suggested I switch to taking the LDN in the morning. Since then I have had no side effects whatsoever.

My initial symptom of numbness on my right side is still there but very mildly, my eyesight did improve quite a lot from the initial damage caused by the neuritis, but since I started taking LDN in June 2015 I have had no relapses and my last MRI showed one diminishing lesion.

My last check-up with the neurologist showed no evident deterioration in my condition. Of course, I will never know whether the disease would have progressed if I had taken nothing, but my quality of life on LDN has been superb, whereas I understand my quality of life had I started on the mainstream drugs would most certainly not be as good.

So, to summarise, since starting LDN I have enjoyed almost eight years of a totally normal life and good health. Thank you!

Letitia, UK – Parkinson's Disease

When I think back now, the first symptom was chronic insomnia which was an indicator of Parkinson's disease but on its own it can be many things or nothing. Not long after that came inexplicable anxiety, something I'd never really had trouble with before. Then gradually more and more symptoms became evident like: constipation, loss of my sense of smell and bladder spasms. I soon noticed tremors in my extremities and left foot drop. I was tripping over things that weren't there and falling upstairs, I was always covered in bruises.

A few months passed like that and then my husband noticed that my arms didn't swing when I walked, he said I looked "wooden". Then came the weakness in my legs, debilitating fatigue and pain and stiffness in my muscles. It was my family who noticed that my voice had gone really quiet and my facial expressions weren't right any more, my face seemed stuck in a severe expression I was told, I had no idea. I couldn't write with ease any more, it seemed I had to fight to control the pen and I lost coordination, even taking something from my pocket turned into a long-drawn-out task that generally failed.

I had to leave work; I was now disabled. After seeing many doctors, I finally got the Parkinson's diagnosis which just seemed like a death sentence to me, a long slow death that would devastate my family.

I was prescribed levodopa, which did help to begin with but after a while it seemed to cause more problems than it was solving. So, the next drug was benztropine which helped with the tremor but I then started having problems remembering things, my short-term memory was terrible. There were other drugs but I was beyond hope by this time and didn't want to try rasagiline coupled with levodopa and whatever else they wanted to mix into the cocktail, I just didn't see the point any more, nothing was helping without causing some other, usually mental, issue and I had enough to deal with.

After much research, helped by my husband, we read about low dose naltrexone and my husband wanted me to try it. It seemed that it wouldn't mush my brain or cause other nasty side effects so I was willing to give it a go. We found the LDN Research Trust website very useful for finding a prescriber, as we knew I would need a private prescription, my neurologist was annoyed with me enough for not simply accepting the drugs I'd been prescribed.

I got my LDN in early 2018 and was taking 1.5 mg for 5 months before increasing to 3 mg and then 4.5 mg. I noticed a feeling of wellbeing, I felt happier and more hopeful, in the first month, the anxiety wasn't such an issue any more. Then gradually, over a period of about a year, all of my symptoms seemed to reverse! Apart from occasional small tremors in my feet and my sense of smell isn't quite what it used to be, but I can smell things now, everything else is good! Not as perfect as if I'd never had these issues for so long but I can function normally now, and I can enjoy life.

I've gone from no hope and severe depression to looking forward to life again and it's incredible! If only I'd been given this drug, this chance for a normal life, back in 2011 when all this was starting – that's a lot of years to lose, feeling hopeless and miserable. But I am grateful that we found it, maybe without all those years of misery I wouldn't fully appreciate the wonderful life I have now. Thank you to the LDN Research Trust for bringing awareness of LDN to all the people needlessly suffering for years.

Anita, USA – Multiple Sclerosis

My name is Anita DiSarli and I live in the United States of America and was diagnosed the year of 2003 with remitting relapsing multiple sclerosis. I started taking LDN the year of 2007 at 4.5 mg a day, which to date is 16 years taking the LDN. I highly recommend anyone diagnosed with multiple sclerosis to try it. I am living proof after many years of taking LDN that it truly works for you and enables you to lead a healthy normal life. Myself personally I would never take anything else. With my sincerity I highly recommend.

KT, USA – Multiple Sclerosis

While I was diagnosed with MS in 2015, now that I know more about the condition, I can trace many symptoms back to the onset of puberty. One of my worst symptoms is spasticity. I hold a lot of tension in my body and often tear muscles and tendons. I would typically experience a fairly major tear three or four times a year, which was very painful and would also significantly limit my physical ability for several months, which in turn, negatively impacted my ongoing sleep, mood, and overall quality of life.

I sustained additional damage in my left leg following a lumbar puncture in 2016 that triggered sciatica and nerve damage from hip to ankle. The sensations were very prominent and always there, which made it very difficult to focus on and enjoy various aspects of life. Beyond the internal nerve pain, even the softest clothing was irritating on my skin. While physical therapy would help significantly with recovery of the muscle and tendon tears, nothing helped the ongoing nerve pain.

I don't recall where I first learned about LDN, but I immediately devoured all the relevant information on the LDN Research Trust website and asked my neurologist about it at my next appointment. He was supportive, although he had never prescribed it before (2021), and I'm happy to say that now he prescribes LDN to many of his patients with success!

I started at 4.5 mg rather than titrating up as I learned on social media that many do. Even though I'm very sensitive to pharmaceuticals and was nervous about not starting lower, I trusted my doctor and I'm glad I did! As far as side effects, the first night my sleep was off - I was awake more than not with a wandering mind, but after that first night my sleep improved tremendously.

About five days in I noticed I hadn't felt the nerve pain in my leg that day - AT ALL! This was a miracle and not something I even thought LDN could help with after living with these ongoing sensations for five years. I thought they were with me for life. So grateful. Beyond that, within three to four months I noticed a major shift in my ability to physically do more. Before I was able to walk only about 4,000 steps a day and it felt like a "have to" - with LDN I can get my 10,000+ steps and actually look forward to exercising as an important part of my morning routine. I've only experienced one major muscle tear since I've been on LDN which is a huge improvement for me.

I'm learning just how important pacing is. Just because I feel like I can do more, I still need to be careful and not overdo it. I'm grateful I'm able to spend more time working in the garden which is very important therapy for me. I'm sleeping better, waking up with the sun so I'm accomplishing more each day, and in general I feel like LDN is helping me live well with MS, maintaining as much functionality as possible and supporting my healthy lifestyle interventions.

LDN has made a noticeable difference in my life. Its gentle impact over time has helped me believe that I can live a good life even with a progressive, incurable condition. I tell everyone about LDN and have friends now using it quite successfully for MS, Lyme, ankylosing spondylitis, long COVID symptoms, and more.

Leslie, USA - Multiple Sclerosis

I am taking LDN for multiple sclerosis. I had a serious MS exacerbation in June 2009. I had been diagnosed with probable MS in 1988 because of a temporary loss of eyesight in one eye. I refused testing to get an official diagnosis of MS in 1988 because my husband and I owned our own business and I did not want the diagnosis of MS to show up on my health records (our insurance payments would have gone up!). And at that time there were no approved drugs for MS. This exacerbation in 2009 was a surprise, since I had not had any symptoms since the temporary loss of eyesight in one eye in the 80s.

Within two weeks of having difficulty walking in 2009, I was admitted to the hospital and put on a week of steroid drips. I was paralyzed from my chest down and was having difficulty breathing. I know now that part of the reason I got steroid drips was to help my lungs. I was in the hospital for a month, a long month attempting to learn how to walk again. I had a wonderful neurologist who made sure I had four hours of PT every day while I was in the hospital.

After that month I came home and started having a PT come to my home. The neurologist insisted that I take Copaxone (one of the five FDA approved drugs in 2009). This was a shot that I needed to administer to myself each day.

A nurse came from the drug company to show me how to administer this shot. The drug company also had two different women from other college towns in the US call me to tell me how they had both been on Copaxone for years, administering a shot every day to themselves. It was interesting to me that the drug company went to the trouble to have these two women call me. They were similar in age and had a similar college degree and lived in college towns, as I do. Fortunately, both women at the end of their calls to me, told me that they were in wheelchairs! Copaxone did not sound like a cure to me or would even give me the outcome I wanted: to be symptom free. The Copaxone shot was also giving me terrible spasms every day when I had the shot. I talked to the neurologist about these spasms and he said I had to continue this approved drug.

I continued with PT. After a month of PT at home, I started going three days a week to a PT facility. Neighbors were driving me to the appointments.

I despised those Copaxone shots so much that I finally called a doctor that is into alternative medicine. He suggested that I read about LDN and if I decided the off-label use of this drug sounded like it might be helpful for me, he would write a prescription. It only took myself and my husband a few hours to read about LDN; we called this alternative doctor back and asked for a prescription. We immediately threw away the needles for the shots and the remaining Copaxone (because of our limited insurance, the Copaxone was costing us a few thousand dollars a month).

I started on the LDN on a Friday night (had a PT session that day), did not have PT again until Monday, and when I walked into PT on Monday, my PT wanted to know what in the world I had done over the weekend that would have made my movement so much better. That is how fast LDN worked for me - almost immediately.

I started with 1.5 mg LDN for two weeks, then 3 mg for two weeks and now I have been on 4.5 mg for the last 14 years! The town where I live has a 10K race every Memorial Day. I have done that race several times since I have been on LDN, run/walking when I was younger, now walking in my 70s.

The only side effect from LDN seems that I do not sleep really well. I do eat as much organic food as I can, and I take a lot of vitamin/ mineral supplements that I have researched and feel make a difference for me. I do pay out of pocket for LDN and it costs me about $35 a month.

My alternative doctor tells me that not everyone has the miraculous results like I did.

I walked into my neurologist's office (the same neurologist who had ordered all the PT) after I started LDN and he wanted to know what I had done to be able to walk so well. I said I had thrown away the Copaxone and was taking LDN. He told me he would no longer be my neurologist.

I am so thankful for LDN and have never looked back!

Emiliano, Italy – Multiple Sclerosis

I have secondary progressive MS. I had the first symptom in 1985. It was very difficult to move, walk and do the daily life activities. They gave me beta interferon and an immune suppressant drug, I had no improvement and continuous worsening.

I discovered the American LDN website and the forum, where I learned about LDN.

My family MD gave me the prescription. I was the first to use LDN in Italy. I started with 1.5 mg and I had no side effects, only two days of insomnia. Nowadays I take 4 mg. I had a lot of improvement after less than one week. The difference between before LDN and after LDN is like if I was born again.

Today I am in contact with more or less all the Italian LDN users, and I can affirm that, about 90% of them have had big improvements.

Andrea, Austria – Multiple Sclerosis

I consider myself lucky that my doctors in Germany discovered quite early on that I had a form of multiple sclerosis (MS). Finding a treatment that helped me, and that I was comfortable with, took more time.

This is my story: in December 2004 I was being treated for back problems, for which I had already had surgery. But now I was having symptoms I was quite sure were not back-related: I couldn't wiggle my toes, and I had trouble climbing stairs. My symptoms moved up my body to the point when lifting my arm to blow dry my hair was more difficult than it had been before.

So, I went to the hospital in December. I had just turned 42. I had an MRI. The doctors were puzzled by what they saw. The MRI showed multiple lesions in my brain; the most active lesion was as big as a golf ball. This explained why my walking and lifting of my arm were impaired to the point where I resembled a stroke patient.

The lumber puncture confirmed I had MS, but all the doctors who saw me and my scans were confused about what kind of MS it was. To this day they still are! But they all agree that it is some form of MS, no matter which terms they use to describe it.

After receiving my first infusion of high-dose steroids, I was able to wiggle my toes and, a bit later, to walk around, though with difficulty. My doctors urged me to start interferon therapy as soon as possible. I did this for two and a half years but had another episode six months later. In large part, though, my symptoms were better with steroids.

While I was still on interferon therapy, I continued to suffer from a slight dropping or stamping of my right foot when I walked. I experienced this during my first episode in 2004. I was able to walk for 20 minutes, but then the weakness would return and I had to rest a bit.

I was not content with this form of therapy - interferon and steroids - or with living this way. So, after two and a half years of once-weekly interferon therapy, I stopped it. The side effects - high fever and flu-like symptoms - had not been pleasant and anyway, I wanted to see what would happen if I went off medication.

After six months I had another episode. This time I had trouble seeing and I was prescribed steroids again. Even though I was still resistant to going back to "mainstream" medication, the steroids did the trick again and I was fine for a while. Another episode followed; this time my speech was affected. Again, steroids helped.

My doctor urged me to start some sort of interferon therapy again. He was afraid that the steroids would lose their magic. I opted not to take the interferon therapy.

I discovered LDN on the internet, LDNinfo.org, and became a member of the low dose naltrexone Yahoo group, where I communicated with many people. With some of them I am still in contact to this day. I printed out all the info I could get and returned to my doctor who diagnosed me in December 2004. He had never heard about LDN but gave me a prescription.

I started LDN in the Spring of 2008, 4.5 mg LDN capsules from a pharmacy in Florida.

When I started LDN in the Spring/Summer of 2008, I recognized in July (after being on LDN for two months) that my foot drop/ weakness was gone. For nine years I did not have any MS episodes or symptoms.

In September 2017 I had another episode with minor motor skills, which I detected quite early, and was put on steroids again, and my symptoms went away. I changed my LDN dose from 4.5 mg to 3 mg and I am doing my best to avoid gluten and cut down on meat.

In Spring 2021, in the middle of the corona epidemic, I got another episode; steroids did the trick again. To this day I am taking 3 mg LDN and unless they find a cure for MS I will continue doing so.

I consider myself very lucky. In the 19 years of MS I have found doctors who were willing to go my way with LDN. I am sure that without the help of the LDN support groups, my story would be different.

Niamh, Ireland – Multiple Sclerosis

I started taking LDN four months after being diagnosed with MS. I could barely get out of bed with fatigue prior to taking it and struggled to walk any distance. As a previously active person who ran regularly it was a significant, unwelcome change.

One week after taking LDN my energy levels improved greatly. The only side effects were unusual dreams the first week and some disrupted sleep but other than that it has been a very positive experience and essentially it has given me the ability to return to work and live life fully.

I have been taking it for ten years now and each year I seem to feel even better. Logically, choosing this medication makes sense to me as there are little to no side effects, it is not a burden on the taxpayer as many medications are, and the effect is very positive.

Pamela, USA – Multiple Sclerosis

Like so many others I went many years without a diagnosis. Many times my symptoms were explained away as anxiety or panic attacks. For a long time I had intermittent issues like walking off balance, issues with my eye, numbness in my extremities and just being downright tired. Having no insurance, I went to a neurologist clinic only to be told that I was "Changing my symptoms and looked disheveled." Needless to say, I became extremely depressed and at one point thought of ending my life.

Having known someone with MS I realized I had many of the same symptoms, but again with no health coverage I could not get an MRI or other testing. During this time I visited numerous MS groups on social media and the internet and LDN was a topic of conversation on many. The more I read, the more I knew that if I was diagnosed that was the medication I would try.

In 2005 I finally had an MRI which showed lesions consistent with MS. The neurologist wanted me on a conventional medication but I was hell-bent on the medication that so many were having great results with, with minimal side effects. After a year and another MRI that "Lit up like a Christmas tree" I printed out information for my neurologist about LDN and he agreed to prescribe it.

I started low dose naltrexone in 2006 and within one week I was less tired, my balance began to improve and my bladder issues lessened.

My new neurologist is now prescribing it for me and she is amazed at how well I'm doing. I am her only patient on it so far. I went from using a cane constantly to walking without one for over two years now. I do take breaks from taking it once in a while either due to it not working as well or finances. But I realize quickly that without LDN my symptoms gradually start to revert to what they used to be. I am 63 years old now and hope to be able to stay on it for life.

Rena, USA - Neuro/Movement Disorder

I developed something called orthostatic tremor at 40. It sounds benign, but makes it difficult for load-bearing joints to withstand the weight of gravity, which means that something as simple as standing to brush my teeth, navigating parking lot obstacles, standing from a sitting position, waiting in line, etc. had become nearly impossible. The muscles cramp and spasm are dystonic, hyper-reflexive, over-producing lactic acid, and my limbs will shake until I feel like falling.

I spent several years on a combination cocktail of anti-epileptics, anticonvulsants, dopaminergics, benzodiazepines, muscle relaxers, pain killers and so much more that were causing significant cognitive impairment, including memory loss. Bilateral DBS implants were installed causing me to feel like I was having a stroke and a seizure every time I turned them on/off.

In 2018, all of my maintenance drugs and "take as needed" drugs combined to create serotonin syndrome turning me into one big painful cramp, with insomnia and an inability to eat much.

I started LDN shortly thereafter, following my research of it for its anti-inflammatory properties, as well as its studied uses on similar neurological conditions (e.g., MS). I had run across a web page managed by a woman in Daytona who has MS and had developed a global database of LDN prescribers, which I have had occasion to provide to some of my other OTers who have tried it.

As expected, my neuro did not initially want to prescribe it. She stated several specific challenges, which I addressed with her:

"That's not what it's for!" She had issue with "off-label" use and/or its primary use for opioid overdoses. I provided research studies.

"We don't know what it will do." She wasn't sure of side effects. I explained it doesn't cause brain or liver damage or renal failure like some of the other drugs I had been on.

At 3 mg, my balance, pain and inflammation were greatly improved. My abdominal cramps did not let up for quite some time, and they had activated various nerves, but the majority of my rigidity quickly diminished.

Initially, the tremor was still bad in my legs. I was spastic. But it was as if all of that rigidity and feeling of heaviness was replaced with rubber and hyper-reactive joints. Note, I also have something called hyperreflexia, so normally, my reflexes are excessive. Regardless, I felt great - a sense of "well-being" much like CBD provides. I still had problems getting around, but it wasn't for a lack of effort or want. I was still pretty non-ambulatory for a few more weeks.

Upon titrating to 4.5 mg, I gradually felt less tremor in my legs and trunk when standing and my standing time had increased to about ten minutes. I was no longer leaning on things to accommodate myself, nor required assistive mobility devices or my DBS anymore.

It's not a cure, but it's a vast improvement with hope for an improved quality of life. The fatigue and the pouring sweat is still real on bad days, but I can now get dressed and conduct basic tasks without "overdoing it." So, it does shift the definition of "strenuous" that this condition forces OTers to live within. It appears to have slowed the diseases progression, at minimum. That said, anecdotally, older OTers who tried it, found little to no success with LDN. So it seems that the earlier in disease progression you start the LDN, the better off you may be.

Sallie, USA – Multiple Sclerosis

At the end of my PhD degree, I was a mess of concerning health problems and received a diagnosis of multiple sclerosis (MS). These symptoms didn't follow the relapsing-remitting course, they just got steadily worse.

I suddenly struggled to spell most words and took ages to write a short email; word finding was slow when speaking; numb hands meant it was difficult to write legibly or wash my hair; my eyes hurt with every movement; I had bladder issues; I needed to hold onto something when standing; my skin was covered in bruises from glancing off furniture or falling over; and walking was difficult due to numbness, drop foot, and ever-present exhaustion. My future looked very limited.

I attended an expensive appointment with someone rated as a top neurologist. They inaccurately took down my health history, despite the summary I had brought along, and offered the same drugs with serious side effects as my local hospital.

My GP at the time suggested I read *Up the Creek with a Paddle* by Mary Boyle Bradley and I also got the newly-published *The LDN Book*. I wanted to try LDN and my GP wrote me a private prescription which I sent to a pharmacy in Glasgow. Initially I bought the liquid to titrate up before switching to the capsules.

LDN instantly halted my frightening downward spiral and gradually improved my symptoms. I experienced no negative side effects at any time. Alongside taking LDN I changed my diet, and used my research skills to create a protocol to support healing.

Despite the delightful effects of LDN, aided by various other lifestyle choices, I had my prescription taken away from me last year. My GP left the practice and no other doctor would write my private prescription. I only rely on the NHS for annual blood tests and have been several years without the need for any other appointments. I appealed to various local medical places and provided factual information about LDN, but could not find a doctor who was prepared to help me. I pay for my prescription and my medicine now.

These days I feel mentally and physically agile and have long been able to return to paid work with a commute that involves walking, a train and two tubes. Thankfully the diagnosis I received for MS six years ago is rarely on my mind. This is primarily due to LDN. I would love it if more people, and pets, were allowed to find out if they could benefit from taking it.

Carol, USA – Multiple Sclerosis

My own journey with MS started when I had dreadful pain in one eye and eventually lost the sight in that eye. That whole attack lasted seven weeks and I was terrified I had a brain tumor. It turned out to be optic neuritis. I went on to have further attacks but the hospital didn't tell me what they thought was wrong! They kept telling me it was all to do with my age and being a woman!

They let me find out myself when I did a search for optic neuritis online and the words multiple sclerosis jumped out of the screen. I was absolutely terrified as all I could imagine was life in a wheelchair and going blind, as each time I had an attack more of my vision was lost.

Over the next few years I had several relapses and began to get other symptoms such as burning sensations, crawling feelings in my legs, neuralgia in my face, clusters of migraines, fatigue, my memory was dreadful and concentration bad, shimmering across my vision, and I went through a spell of tripping up.

After refusing many times I was talked into trying Rebif injections three times a week - I ended up covered in bruises, feeling extremely tired, and my eyesight was awful. I was eventually told the Rebif was damaging my liver so after a year of injecting I stopped.

I was then told my only other option was to go on Copaxone, injecting every day. I checked out side effects online and was really scared by what I read. I decided there must be something else out there and began trawling the net for an acceptable alternative and that's when I found LDN. I went back to my neurologist and told him that I wanted to try it and I think he could see how determined I was as he agreed to give me a private prescription.

I have now been using the liquid form of LDN since the beginning of July 2012 and I feel great. I have settled on taking 3 mg each day, as when I increased the dose I had awful headaches and felt like I had flu. I now feel fitter, concentration is better, memory has improved, sleep is better than it has been for years, the shimmering across my vision has gone, and almost all the tingling burning and neuralgia seem to have stopped (don't want to speak too soon and am touching wood as I write this, but after all this time I'm pretty sure it will last).

I have also been discharged from the hospital eye department as my vision seems to have stabilized. In fact, the consultant said my sight has actually improved! I still have days when I feel exhausted but these tend to be when I have been away for a weekend with friends or when I have had to deal with something stressful, but with lots of rest I bounce back.

I would say to anyone thinking of trying LDN to go for it. It really has changed my health for the better. Good luck to everyone who is just starting out.

Francie, USA - Multiple Sclerosis

I was diagnosed with multiple sclerosis in September 2000, but like everybody else, I had it long before that diagnosis. I think that the worst part was the fatigue. I would go in the back room of my office and lie down on the carpet in the afternoons, and practically not be able to get up.

When I was finally diagnosed, the doctor told me two things about MS. It is progressive and it is incurable, and I found both of those true as long as I used the biologics that they prescribed. The one that I took the longest was Copaxone. It was chosen as the safest treatment, with the least side effects. What I was not told was that according to the research, it was no cure. It was shown to "help" delay progression in only 32% of the people who took it. This is a medication that requires a shot in the stomach every day at the cost of $5,600 per month.

I was obviously among the 68% who got no benefit, but since I did not know of these statistics, I continued to take that shot daily for over nine years, while rapidly going downhill. By 2006, I was mostly in a wheelchair and nearly bed bound from the MS. The Texas heat was so debilitating, that we bought a ranch in Kentucky to try to live a better life. It really did not help, since I would still get overheated by wearing a coat in the winter, when we would go in a building I could not take it off rapidly enough.

By 2009, I had lost my job and with it, my health insurance, and that is when I found out what the insurance had been paying for the worthless treatment that I had been given. A whopping $5,600 per month! For a couple of months, I bought the Copaxone off of a neighbor who had also not found any benefit from it. We paid her enough for her car payment, but even that was more than we could afford after losing my job. I had to admit defeat and felt sure that there was no hope of having a life with MS.

Six months later, I had finally read enough on the internet to decide to give the LDN a try. I had probably heard about it as much as two years before, but for some reason, it just did not click. I believed in my doctors, not some snake oil. But I had run out of options and it seemed like it was worth a try. I contacted my neurologist, and asked her to prescribe it for me. Her answer was a flat "No."

I finally started to understand that our medical system is involved with keeping people sick and on expensive treatments, not actually curing a disease. There is no additional money to be had when you cure a disease, but developing a treatment designed to keep the patient on a treatment long term, has huge benefits to the doctors and pharmaceutical companies.

I eventually managed to get a prescription for naltrexone, though not from my neurologist. Then I talked my dear husband, Chuck, into being my guinea pig and control subject. If he took it too, I would know if what I was feeling was from the LDN or something else entirely. Chuck had allergies so he also got a prescription at the same time.

We started May 1, 2009. I still think of it as my second birthday, when I got my life back.

Back then, everybody started at 3 mg and went to 4.5 when they felt like it. So, we both started at 3 mg. I woke up that first morning with a totally different attitude. I felt like I finally had some energy and a happier outlook. Over the next 18 months, things continued to improve along with losing nearly 70 pounds. I was an addictive eater and was also immobile. I started to move and exercise more. I started to cook better food, and my food cravings disappeared as the endorphins increased, which is often what causes addictive eating in the first place (lack of endorphins).

About a year later, I was diagnosed with uterine cancer that obviously predated the start of my LDN. It is very difficult for medications and the immune system to get to the inside of the uterus. We were ranchers and I no longer had health insurance. The estimate from the University of Kentucky was $35,000 to $50,000. I said, "I can get my dog spayed for 200 bucks, what are you doing with the other $49,000?" Zip! Right over their heads. They had no answer. We turned to medical tourism and contacted the doctors that we thought would help. The organization we contacted works with international doctors to make sure that you are getting the best care. A radical hysterectomy was $4,500 including a bilingual liaison to get us to doctors visits, the store, the pharmacy or any place else that we needed. The facilities in Mexico were absolutely state of the art, since there is universal health care in Mexico and the facilities are provided by the government.

I credit the LDN with helping me to survive the maximum dose radiation and chemo treatments, that would have eliminated my immune system without it. After radiation and chemo, there was nothing left that they could do, so they turned me over to hospice and went on to their next victims.

Once again, I hit the internet for research and found a number of treatments that were designed to build health, not directly cure disease. I used off-the-shelf treatments to eliminate parasites and fungus and I fasted to starve the fast-reproducing cancer cells. I used LDN of course as well as alpha-lipoic acid. I went from hospice to full remission and have stayed cancer free for over ten years now, with the same simple products.

One of the biggest treats was that Chuck's horrible allergy to poison ivy went away (remember he was my "control subject"). We live on a ranch, so this over-the-top reaction can be really debilitating. It did not seem to happen the first summer, probably because we were not looking for it, but by the second summer, he could play in the stuff. He has remained free of any allergies for the 14 years since starting LDN in 2009. Sometimes he is a bigger advocate than I am.

Cameon, USA – Multiple Sclerosis

After learning of and researching LDN, I requested it from my GP because my MS was worsening, and I was headed for a nursing home. He knew of full dose naltrexone and was willing to prescribe low dose naltrexone for me. He gave me a prescription for 5 mg, which was higher than I'd read about, but I figured I could always lower it if needed.

I was very apprehensive to take it, scared of what I had read about possible side effects, but I put on my "big girl" panties and swallowed the capsule! My LDN journey had begun. The rest, as they say, is history!

In order to realize just how much LDN has improved my quality of life, prior to LDN, here's how I described my existence: sitting in a wheelchair living inside a paint shaker which was on a moving merry-go-round with a jello floor, watching a 1950's home movie.

Within the first few weeks, I experienced both improvements and side effects. The internal paint shaker had all but shut off, but I did have stomach aches, headaches, hot flashes and periodic insomnia. In experimenting, I changed the filler from Avicel to ginger, and the dosing time from night to morning, then to 1:00 p.m., and eliminated all those issues.

Along with the paint shaker all but eliminated, or perhaps because of it, I saw an increase in strength, balance and energy. My fine motor skills improved and I forced myself, successfully, to rely less on the grab bars I used when transferring from my wheelchair.

About eight months into taking LDN, I experienced a "lull" in improvement, so I skipped a dose, as I had read sometimes receptors needed to be reset. Definitely not for me! All the old symptoms returned.

However, two months after skipping a dose, just ten short months after starting LDN, using an upright walker, I walked into the adjustment room at my chiropractor's! That was in July of 2019. Since then, I have happily left the chair in the vehicle at the chiropractor's and used only the walker! My chiropractor even told me that I didn't feel as "mushy". So, was the skipping helpful or was it the exercising, walker therapy, increased strength, energy and balance? Most likely, a combination of them all.

One night I even stood upright, making certain my balance was stable, and purposely took the TWO small steps required to get to my bed, totally unassisted!

The paint shaker has stopped, the merry-go-round is mainly at a stand-still, concrete has replaced the jello flooring, and the home movie has ended.

I noticed improvements other than walking. For instance, my speech isn't nearly as slurred as it was. I used to be out of breath so much more often than I am now, and I no longer suffer with unruly sinuses.

LDN has been called a game changer and a life saver. It certainly was for me. I am no longer nursing home bound, thanks to God and LDN!

Angela, Australia – Multiple Sclerosis

I was diagnosed with multiple sclerosis 12 years ago. My neurologist gave me a load of information about treatment options, none of which I wanted as my body was already burdened with reactions to failed treatments for wrong diagnoses over the previous three years. I was suffering from urticaria, severe fatigue and adrenal failure, pain, tremor and brain fog - these on top of my MS symptoms, or maybe some were MS symptoms as it progressed while being treated for the wrong things. I was also taking temazepam for insomnia as that was just adding more misery to an already miserable existence.

The symptoms that sent me to see my doctor in the first place, around 2008, were vision problems accompanied by loss of balance and dizziness and occasional tremors. All the rest, including the bladder issues and relentless pain, came on over the years of misdiagnosis and varying drug treatments. It wasn't neuropathy, it wasn't Parkinson's, it wasn't just a random autoimmune disease that required DMARDs or biologics. It was MS, and that hit me hard because this neurologist did extensive tests, more so than any other, and he eliminated all the previous diagnoses and I knew that that was it.

So when the neurologist, who had earned my trust with his thoroughness and caring attitude, started talking about LDN I listened. I was wary, I was sick of drugs and the additional problems they all seemed to come with. I went home and talked to my husband and he researched low dose naltrexone and he was very positive about it. I went back to the neurologist and agreed to try it.

He started me on a very low dose, being considerate of my sensitivities. I increased the dose slowly over months until I got to 5 mg. I tried 6 mg but that seemed to not work the same as 5 mg. I tried 4 mg and that also didn't feel as good as 5. So 5 mg was my happy dose. My health significantly improved as the months went on. The pain subsided, the tremors stopped, my bladder was stronger - no more embarrassing leaking. I could move better, easier. My balance issues just disappeared.

I still have limitations as I had this horrible illness a long time before finding a treatment that would put it in remission but I'm better. And my immune system is better too - I caught COVID last year and overcame it without a vaccine (I wasn't about to subject myself to the uncertainties of that given my history of reactions to drugs).

I'm 63 in November and I'm living with energy, hope, a clear head and the ability to do most of the things I could do before this awful journey started. LDN should be the first drug offered to people with these types of conditions, not the last. It's cheap, it's efficacious and it does no harm, unlike most other pharma drugs offered today. I am eternally grateful to have found a rheumatologist who knew about LDN and was prepared to offer it. I wish all doctors would educate themselves about LDN. It would save a lot of patients an awful lot of misery and pain.

Pat, USA – Multiple Sclerosis

I have multiple sclerosis. I was diagnosed 15 years ago. I have been on LDN for two years. I notice more energy and I have relief of pain from muscle spasms. If I forget to take my LDN I notice a difference.

I currently take Lexapro, Lyrica for PHN, Prevacid. I had no side effects from taking LDN. I have not had a problem getting an LDN prescription. I am not currently on any disease-modifying medications. I feel LDN has helped improve my quality of life.

Donna, USA – Multiple Sclerosis

After several years of various testing, I was lumped into the "fibromyalgia syndrome" diagnosis bag until a neurologist at the Mayo Clinic decided to test me for MS. In the early 1990s, after a battery of tests, including an MRI of my brain, I was diagnosed with remitting and relapsing MS by the Mayo Clinic in Jacksonville, FL. My symptoms ranged from falling down the stairs, tripping over curbs and falling, stuttering, numbness on the right side of my body, unable to brush my hair due to the pain, double vision - the list goes on. After a year of denying my diagnosis, I decided to try the medications that were available at that time. After a short period of time, I stopped the medication and learned to deal with my symptoms because I could not deal with the side effects of the prescribed meds.

During this time, my husband was called about investing in clinical trials for a drug called LDN. As he began to learn more about studies being done at Penn State University for Crohn's disease, he learned that LDN had shown some promising studies for other autoimmune diseases. He began to search for a doctor to prescribe it. It took a while because nobody was interested in reading the studies. Finally, we convinced my psychiatrist to write the prescription. I will admit that I was a sceptic but I agreed to put the pill in my pill box and take it every night.

About three months later, I woke one morning to a feeling I had not felt in a very long time. It was as if the lights came on! My energy levels increased, the pain was less, I stopped falling as much, I actually felt pretty good for the first time in a long time! I took me a while to put two and two together - IT MUST BE THE LDN!!

I have been taking LDN for approximately 30 years, only stopping for a few surgeries. I am 72 and I rarely get sick. No COVID until 2022, but it was a mild case while all my family were very sick and have had several bouts. We have three great-grandchildren who pick up every germ. It seems like everyone in the family gets sick - but not me! I believe 4.5 mg/nightly has boosted my immune system but, more importantly, it keeps my MS under control. My primary care doctor is amazed but will not read the literature that I have shared with him about LDN, causing me to change doctors. I get my medication from a compounding pharmacy, still being prescribed by my psychiatrist who, incidentally, prescribes it for many of his patients.

I have told anyone who will listen about LDN. Every doctor, nurse, medical professionals in my family who have watched me live with MS, friends…everyone. I have even watched a miraculous benefit from LDN when our dog sitter began to get sick. She went from a very active person to a wheel chair in a matter of a few months, diagnosed with progressive MS. I told her about LDN and how it helped me. She told her doctor who was willing to let her try it. The doctor actually called me to hear my story and to see what the side effects were in my experience. She began taking LDN. We didn't see her for a while. When we needed a dog sitter, we called to see how she was doing and to see if her daughter could sit for us. To our surprise, she showed up to sit for our dog. Instead of a wheelchair, she showed up in yoga pants and joggers! Even more importantly, she was training for a walk/run marathon, in which she participated a few weeks later!!

I believe LDN has saved my life. It makes me angry that most doctors will not even listen to my story nor will they read the studies and literature that I share with them.

My grandson is a doctor of nursing, specializing in lung cancer and he thinks it is hype. His wife runs an infusion clinic where she administers MS IV drugs every day and she will not listen, even though she knows it is compounded and prescribed every day for pediatric Crohn's disease.

LDN has added years to my life. I am grateful that more and more medical professionals are recognizing its benefits. Thank you to the LDN Research Trust for all the work they do to inform people of this marvelous drug. I pray that more and more people will become aware and that medical professionals will read the studies and give it a try for their patients. If one day, this pill could be produced instead of compounded, that might encourage more doctors to try it.

Yvonne, UK – Dystonia

I take LDN for dystonia. I had a form of lockjaw for which I tried many medications prescribed by my doctor. I also tried many forms of relaxation, mindfulness, chiropractors, meditation, acupuncture, the list goes on. The only thing that worked was my LDN. It has been a miracle worker.

I literally could not open my mouth at one point to eat. I survived on liquids.

This illness came on very suddenly. The doctor was unsure of the treatment I needed. It was all trial and error to no effect. My son had researched LDN and we felt it was worth a try. It was truly a miracle worker for me.

I have now been taking LDN for more than five years. It gave me back my confidence and health and my life came back to normality.

SKIN CONDITIONS

Tam, USA – Lichen Sclerosus

I am a 65-year-old woman who has suffered from lichen sclerosus since adolescence. It is an autoimmune skin disease of genitals. Needless to say, it can be catastrophic to one's sexual health, cause terrible childbirth complications and great shame. Few doctors are familiar with it but little research has been done.

The treatment includes using very strong corticosteroids, strong topical corticosteroids (clobetasol) to prevent cancer. The side effects from the clobetasol include thinning of skin and eventual loss of vulvar architecture.

I heard about LDN being researched as a treatment for psoriatic arthritis, which I have also recently been diagnosed with. I found the patient support groups on Reddit and social media and decided to try it with the blessing of my rheumatologist.

My starting dose, just six weeks ago, was 0.5 mg and I have titrated up to 1 mg, taken at bedtime. It has helped with more restful sleep at night, mood, clarity of thought and moderately with joint pain.

Most miraculous is the healthy pink skin now appearing where the thick white lichen patches were. I am cautiously optimistic that this is the answer I have been searching for for decades. I would love for lichen sclerosus patients to find out about LDN to see if it might help others.

Shannon, USA - Granuloma Annulare (GA)

In October of 2020 (pre-COVID vaccine!) I noticed a rash on my lower legs that resembled a flea bite attack (small spots but more than 50 on each leg). The spots did not itch or hurt initially. I had waxed my lower legs the month before and most of the spots were where I had waxed. More appeared on my feet and hands and a couple on my thighs and elbows. The spots on my hands and feet got thick and rubbery and over a few years, the individual spots on the huge outbreak on my legs began to spread out and join each other.

Around April or May of 2021, I went to the dermatologist who did a biopsy and confirmed that I had a stubborn autoimmune disease, granuloma annulare (GA) that was very hard to get rid of and should not be painful or itchy - just ugly and likely would "go away in a few years...". They said it was rare and went along with my late onset of type 1 diabetes (eight years ago, when I was 54). The doctor sent me home with sticky cortisone skin-thinning creams and later tried shooting Kenalog into some of the bigger spots - that made my blood sugars high.

I moisturized constantly over the year and exfoliated with brushing, tried applying apple cider vinegar, peroxide, no dairy or gluten, pre and probiotics, many vitamins and supplements, tried infrared light, spent close to $1,000 on things that folks suggested from the social media support group that has more than 9,000 of us, many plagued with GA for over 40 years!

The GA on my legs began to be painful especially at night - like my legs were wrapped in jellyfish! I spent hours a day doing things to my legs and researching for myself. I was offered a cocktail of five "biologic" antibiotics that might work in 6 to 12 months. Depression ensued plus osteoarthritis really flared in my back last summer (2022) through the fall.

In February I began taking LDN after a couple of GA support group friends said they thought it was working, but not until 6 to 12 months. I was able to get it from an on-line pharmacy after answering some health questions. My primary care doctor approved of it and was prescribing it for a fibromyalgia patient.

I started at 1.5 mg for ten days, then 3 mg for a few weeks and finally up to 4.5 where I have stayed. I did have terribly painful sleep for a year and a half before I began LDN so the dreaming symptom (which still happens sometimes) did keep me up at first. I was originally taking it at bedtime but have found that taking it during the day is better for me.

After several months at 4.5 mg I definitely noticed more energy, less back pain, less nerve pain in my leg skin, less peeling of the skin and now at six and a half months the skin on my legs is changing to a marbled look. It is still a little sensitive and it is not pretty but I have so much hope. The inflammation is dissipating.

I believe LDN is harmless - I have not been sick since I have been taking LDN. I want to keep taking it indefinitely, even when/if my GA clears. LDN means hope for me.

Patricia, UK – Psoriasis and Psoriatic Arthritis

I can't remember when the psoriasis first showed itself, I was in my teens, I'm 42 now – so I've had it for roughly 25-30 years. It started on my knees and that's when the doctor diagnosed it as psoriasis. It didn't spread though, it just stayed on my knees, was irritating and I kept my knees covered because it didn't look nice. I was prescribed different creams and none of them did anything so I stopped bothering and just kind of accepted it as one of life's little irritations.

It stopped being merely irritating when I was in my early twenties, when it started to spread to my thighs and then appeared on my elbows and forearms. Now I had to cover my arms too. I was prescribed pretty much the same creams, which hadn't improved over the years. I kept applying the creams and the psoriasis continued to spread to my lower legs and upper arms. That went on for a few years until it became infected. Once it's infected it just spreads like wildfire. This is when the pain started, the pain in my joints.

I was referred to a specialist who diagnosed psoriatic arthritis too. I was losing my eternal optimism and I'd stopped any kind of acceptance of my situation at this point. I've always been a really positive person, there's always someone worse off than yourself – but I was beginning to feel that this was unfair, I didn't deserve this. The itch was painful, it's hard to describe to someone who hasn't experienced it, there are no descriptive words that adequately cover the sensation. If I said burn, prickly – like hundreds of stabbing needles – you still couldn't grasp how horrible it is.

And, if anything can be worse; the unsightliness of it, the way people wanted to pull back if you passed them something – they didn't want to touch my hand because it looked like I had some kind of plague or something. It doesn't do a lot for your self-confidence. It made my life really miserable. It certainly dictated my wardrobe.

I eventually went for phototherapy treatment. First ultraviolet B, which slows the production of skin cells, and I had to go 3 times a week for 6 weeks. It worked, the psoriasis started to go and by the end of two months it had all but cleared. I was elated! But 10 months later it started to come back and it was savage, it was worse than before. It was all over my arms, legs, torso and it started to come up on my face. I just wanted to hide away and die. The dermatologist was offering me methotrexate and biologics but I didn't want those, they mess with your immune system in a negative way and I was already struggling with a messed up immune system, if they couldn't actually fix my immune system, I didn't want them messing with it further.

I was back on the waiting list to try psoralen plus ultraviolet A. I waited 8 months for the appointment. I was given a tablet containing psoralen, which, it was explained to me, makes the skin more sensitive to light. Yes it did that. I burned. I itched, I had headaches – each time I went. And this treatment can cause skin cancer, more so than the other because of the psoralen.

It started to work; the redness was fading. Then my life went all upside down, I lost my job, my father had a heart attack and it was just so stressful. This, mid-way through treatment, was the catalyst for a body wide break out. I honestly just wanted to crawl away and die. With all the stress and worry and the pain of my skin crawling, and my joints feeling like they were full of broken glass, - I was just overwhelmed.

I looked horrific; I knew I did. I didn't want to go out, I didn't want people looking at me and thinking I was some diseased plague victim or something. The pains were getting worse too, in my knees, ankles and wrists. I was taking pain killers like they were going out of fashion.

Spending lots of time indoors now, and having lost my job, it was easy for me to become a bit of a hermit – I didn't have to put a brave face on it anymore and I just lost all confidence. So I spent a lot of time on the internet. I wish I'd done it earlier instead of relying on doctors and dermatologists, that was a complete waste of time that I could have been living! It comes down to the fact that you pass responsibility for your health and happiness to someone else, a doctor, and you don't take responsibility for yourself. Bad health isn't something you should be passive about.

Having all that time alone I ventured into help groups online, other people also felt like I did and looked like I did. Why didn't I do this before?

This is where I found people talking about low dose naltrexone, or LDN as it's known. I was interested because so many said that it had helped them, a few said it didn't but more said that it had. I gathered all the information I could find and took it to my doctor. I told him that nothing that he had done, or the dermatologist had done, had helped me so I wanted to try LDN. Amazingly – he said no! How could he say no when all the stuff he'd given me had failed? He wasn't even interested in looking at the information I'd taken. I was stunned that he should be so dismissive.

Okay, I thought, I'll buy it from abroad, I'd seen a link for that – though it was worrying because it's dodgy, to say the least, but I was past caring at this point. It was while I was searching for that link that I came across the LDN Research Trust website and they had lists of prescribers for those who wanted to go private. I found my nearest prescriber and arranged a consultation and it was so straight forward I was a bit taken aback.

I got my LDN a week later through the post. It was that simple. I just needed to provide proof of diagnosis and have a chat on the phone with a doctor. I could have done this years ago and I grieve for those years that needn't have been so awful.

That was 5 years ago and I'm still on LDN now, always will be. I started at 4.5 mg and had no issues, other than more realistic dreams, which were actually pleasant. I noticed in the first month how much better I felt in myself, in spite of the painful, itchy skin and joint pains. Then the joint pains reduced to nothing by the end of around 6 weeks. I noticed my skin not feeling so sensitive to the touch of my clothing and by 3 months the horrible scaliness of my skin was less silvery, less rough. It just got better and better.

The big patches just reduced in size and faded and by 9 months, around there, I was seeing lots more pink skin with occasional patches of dryness. Now of course I have pink skin, smooth skin and I can wear sleeveless tops and I got my social life back. I am so happy that it's finally gone. My confidence increased as the horrible looking skin decreased and I found another job. And my father is fine by the way, he recovered really well.

LDN should be offered as a first line treatment for autoimmune skin conditions, we should be given the choice. I share my story as often as I get the chance now, nobody should have to suffer like that for decades, and when standard treatments clearly aren't working then doctors should look elsewhere and be interested enough to take notice when a patient suggests something that they've found.

Don't waste time like I did, read about LDN and get a consultation, you won't lose anything by trying it but it might just give you your life back.

Michele, UK – Painful Undiagnosed Rash

My skin went nuts in March 2019. I had bumps and redness first on my hands. It then spread to my arms, chest, breasts, stomach and then my inner thighs which erupted like a volcano and the pain was the worst I have ever known, and I have given birth and been burnt. I could hardly walk.

My GP put me on steroids which did not help. I was put in hospital and the nurses thought I had had acid thrown at my thighs. I was on 90 mg of steroids a day, then they wanted to put me on the drugs that they give transplant patients, despite them being unable to give a diagnosis. The assumption is that it was an autoimmune issue of some unknown nature.

My husband did not want me on those drugs and after researching we discovered LDN. I had been trying to reduce the steroids by 10 mg a week but when I started LDN at 0.25 mg I found I could reduce the steroids and eventually came off them altogether. We get the prescription from a private doctor and send it to Scotland to get it filled. I started taking LDN in the last weeks of August and was so much better by the end of September. My skin is fine now.

Both my husband and I now take LDN. We alternate the dose daily. I take 2 mg one day, 1.5 mg the next, then 1 mg the next and 0.5 mg the next day and so on. My husband takes the same doses that I do, following the same schedule, just to stay healthy. I also do the intermittent fasting 16/8 and I do a 37 hour fast once a week.

I am 67, I work over 60 hours a week and I feel great and I don't look my age. LDN is wonderful.

Mariana, USA - Psoriasis

I was diagnosed with psoriasis in April 2022. The prescribed medication from my dermatologist was clobetasol, triamcinolone for the body and ketoconazole and fluocinonide for the scalp. Over the course of four months following the above treatment, my condition got worse: I had lost big patches of my hair, got more lesions on my scalp and body, the overall inflammation got worse and out of control.

I had also visited a dermatologist, a specialist in psoriasis, who prescribed me Tremfya and Duobrii, both medications not covered by my medical insurance plan. Not only was I not able to pay their cost of approximately. $14,000/month but I was terrified of their potential side effects which include additional skin problems, respiratory infections, joint pain among many others.

In August 2022, I was blessed to have one of my friends, who had just heard of my health issues, tell me about LDN. For the next two weeks I watched numerous documentaries and video clips about LDN, read *The LDN Book* (first volume) and also, I have found extremely informative, the LDN Research Trust website from where I have found a prescriber and a compound pharmacy in my city to prescribe and provide me with LDN.

By the end of August, I had started with LDN titration (at 0.5 mg up to 4.5 mg). In about two and a half months the skin inflammation started to subdue and by November I noticed the hair started to grow, the lesions were dry and less.

In January 2023 I had 95% of my body and scalp cleared from lesions or any signs of inflammation. Right now, I still continue with the 4.5 mg dose. I am very happy and enjoying my life! Thank you for giving me so much information through the website and newsletters. It was like giving me my life back!

THYROID CONDITIONS

Jen, USA – Graves' Disease

I was diagnosed with Graves' disease in the ER on June 12th, 2022. My symptoms were extreme overheating, brain fog/disconnect, extreme weight loss, extreme hair loss, extreme dry, itchy, scaly, skin, bowel issues - constipation/diarrhea continually, thyroid eye disease, mood swings, extreme fatigue; and I was unable to even drive my car, I had tremors so bad.

I was given methimazole first. I took it for two weeks and developed fast weight gain that would not come off and facial swelling so I stopped. I then was given propylthiouracil (PTU). I also was given propranolol. PTU and propranolol helped alleviate my severe tremors. I had lost bowel control at the time that I was diagnosed and the PTU helped relieve the bowel incontinence. Propranolol helped reduce my heart rate into a normal range most of the time.

After being on PTU for about a month I was able to get off of the propranolol. PTU didn't ever seem to get my numbers in range for my Graves' disease. It did seem to get some symptoms under control but I felt worse than ever, even though some of my symptoms were alleviated.

I heard about LDN from a pharmacy on social media. I happen to have a primary care physician who was familiar with LDN and prescribed it easily for me. I started at 1.5 mg, I am now at 4 mg.

When I first began LDN, I had a pretty bad headache that lasted for about three days, but seemed to get under control with ibuprofen. I had frequent urination for about the first week, and it seemed to taper off. Each time I titrate up, I seem to have a small headache and frequent urination. Those side effects seem to dissipate within a few days.

From the very first dose of LDN at 1.5 mg, I have never had another overheating issue. My hair has completely stopped falling out; I went from hands full of hair in the shower, to three or four hairs when showering. I no longer have brain fog or disconnect.

My weight is normal and balanced. My bowels are regulated and I do not suffer from diarrhea or constipation any longer. My mood has stabilized, and I find myself continually having positive thoughts and feeling hopeful.

My skin all over my entire body feels like baby skin. Even the bottom of my feet are no longer calloused. I have energy every day all day. My fatigue is completely gone. I have cut my PTU in half. My labs are very close to being in range. LDN has given me my life back. I no longer suffer from any Graves' disease symptoms at all.

Nicola, UK – Hashimoto's

I had extreme fatigue, low mood, brain fog and weight gain from 2016. I consulted my GP about pins and needles in my hand and had a blood test which confirmed hypothyroidism. I was then given thyroxine which brought my TSH level back to normal. However, after a year I still did not feel much better and after further tests my GP suggested vitamin supplements and counselling for my mild depression.

After another year or so I was still not feeling much better but because my tests showed as normal the GP was unable to suggest anything else. I had asked about receiving T3 as I knew other people had found this useful and my GP agreed to an appointment with an endocrinologist. I had further tests done but was not prescribed T3 and it was only at this stage I found out it was the autoimmune disorder Hashimoto's and my thyroid antibodies were very high. I still had many of the symptoms and was struggling at work due to fatigue and low mood. This also affected my social and family life.

It seemed to me to be important to tackle the autoimmune problem rather than the symptoms but the medical professionals I have seen do not seem to agree or are not aware of treatments. I did my own research and found the thyroid pharmacist, Mark Ryan and Thyroid UK particularly useful. I changed my diet but this alone was not enough to reduce my symptoms.

Thyroid UK website had useful information about LDN and I really thought it was worth a try. I went direct to a chemist in Glasgow and was able to get a private prescription. I read all the information about LDN so I was aware of how it works and any possible side effects.

I started on a dose of 1.5 mg and worked up to 4.5 mg. After the first month I felt much more energetic and more cheerful. I had occasional headaches and a feeling a bit like a hangover at times. I also had weird and vivid dreams but none of these side effects were persistent or caused me a problem.

There were ups and downs and it seemed quite a gradual process of slowly feeling back to my normal self. After a year I definitely felt back to my previous energy levels, I could get lots done in a day, I felt like exercising, socialising and going out. I had already taken early retirement because I was finding it hard to cope with work. LDN has allowed me to enjoy my life and make the most of it.

I still need to take thyroxine but I have stayed on the same dose since I started which I see as a sign that my thyroid is not deteriorating.

My GP will not test for thyroid antibodies so I am not sure if this has improved. I still have issues with the GP if I have other health problems as on two occasions, I have been advised to stop taking LDN. I would really like to see more awareness of LDN in GP practices as a way of helping many conditions that have limited success with more conventional medication.

Jennifer, USA – Hashimoto's Thyroiditis

My symptoms began in 2005. I worked full time plus taught ten fitness classes weekly with energy to spare prior to my Hashimoto's diagnosis. All of a sudden, I could barely walk upstairs and needed four-hour naps daily. Getting on thyroid meds for the associated hypothyroidism helped, but I still had chronic muscle pain and severe pain/fatigue flares after exercise. Sometimes the pain was so bad I could not sit up at my desk to work. I tried numerous pain meds and muscle relaxants, but none helped. Massage helped pain somewhat but not the post-exercise flares.

I did not learn about LDN until 2020, when I joined an online patient support group. It took me another year to find a physician that would prescribe it. A rheumatologist and my primary care physician had never heard of it.

I was prescribed 1.5 mg, titrating to 3 mg, then 4.5 mg, every three weeks. Initially, I took it nightly as prescribed, but it gave me horrible insomnia. I switched to mornings and now have no side effects.

It took me about three months into the 4.5 mg dose to feel any significant benefit, but now it is literally life-changing! No post exercise pain/fatigue flares, and almost no daily chronic pain for the first time in 15 years! I call LDN "my magic pill." I can't believe I suffered that long in pain!

Sarah, USA – Hashimoto's and TMJ

After my first pregnancy I knew something wasn't right. They didn't catch that I was in a thyroid storm then. After my second pregnancy they diagnosed me in a thyroid storm and then Hashimoto's. I have had it since 2007. TMJ started becoming a very real problem around 2018. The pain was very hard to live with.

My Hashimoto's was very hard to control. Between going to endocrinologists, who wouldn't treat very real symptoms or even listen to me, and doctor after doctor who were all the same as the last, I was losing hope. My jaw pain dictated what I could chew and eat, I bought a very expensive mouth guard which wasn't as much help as I expected and I used lots of heat and ice to try easing the pain.

I was eventually given Botox for the TMJ and levothyroxine daily for Hashimoto's and migraine medication to take as needed.

I heard about LDN when it was first starting to appear on the scene. I didn't want to try it until my nurse practitioner said I should give it a chance. I started LDN in August 2022 on a starting dose of 1.5 mg, going up to 4.5 mg which I take now.

I had an uncommon side effect which was that my taste for coffee completely changed once starting LDN, that lasted maybe six months but I'm back to normal now and enjoy coffee again. I also lost a few pounds in weight but I'd also gone gluten free during the same period so it may have been that. Now I have no side effects whatsoever.

I noticed improvements in my health very quickly, about a month later. My blood sugar seemed more stable, and my anxiety seemed better after a couple months. The pain in my jaw has taken about eight months to ease off and I'm so happy now that I don't have to live with that anymore.

I still take levothyroxine and occasional migraine medication but LDN has made me feel better than I felt ten years ago in my mid 30s. I feel great, so it has felt like it's given me my life back. I have had comments that my body doesn't look "puffy" anymore and I believe my thyroid numbers are better from taking it. I am so glad it was suggested to me.

Marcia, USA – Autoimmune Thyroid Disorder

In the spring of 2022, I noticed my energy level was waning, so I discussed this with my GP and naturopath. I was sent to an endocrinologist. After having radiated iodine scans and a thyroid blood panel, I found out I had no mass, but the T3, T4 and TSH numbers were way higher than normal.

My naturopath had me do a thyroglobulin antibody test, which showed very high results in October, 2022. At this time I was diagnosed with autoimmune thyroid disorder. My naturopath prescribed 0.5 mg naltrexone in October, 2022.

I gradually worked up to 3 mg of naltrexone per day since the beginning of February. I have to break up the dosage, because of vivid dreams keeping me awake at night. However, my March 2023 blood work shows close to normal T3, T4 numbers, and the thyroglobulin results have also improved since October.

The TSH numbers have improved slightly over time. I see my naturopath this week to get her reaction to the results shown in the blood work.

MULTIPLE AUTOIMMUNE CONDITIONS

Kristen Burris, LAc, MSTOM, Dip Acu, USA

At my worst, I was sleeping 12 to 14 hours in the evenings and when I would arise, I had a very difficult time standing to shower. Several times a week I needed a three or four hour nap after work and was horizontal, on a bed or couch, all day long, four days a week.

My postural orthostatic tachycardia syndrome (POTS) would skyrocket my heartrate to 170 upon standing; I'd get breathless and dizzy- just from standing up. I would need a seat to support my lifeless body as I ambled into the shower and remained seated during my showers. The simple act of washing my hair caused extraordinary exhaustion and arm pain and weakness. I'd retreat back to my bed - spent. I'd wrap my wet hair in a towel and pass out for another hour or two. Just a shower did this to my body. The action of pulling a sheet up and over my body was excruciatingly painful. My husband would often report that I sadly moaned from pain while asleep.

The attempt to make the bed and the exertion from showering would require an hour's rest to recover enough so I could work. At work I could no longer stand, as I had for the last 15 years in practice and four years in traditional Chinese medical school. I needed a doctor's stool to sit on and roll around while I treated patients. At my lowest point, after years of missing out, I was researching buying a wheelchair so I could re-engage with life, albeit seated. But I was sick of the years of being 60-80 % bedridden and being unable to go anywhere or do anything.

I would ask every one of my doctors if they thought this was a good idea. Frustratingly, they always said absolutely not. I never pushed them why they answered that way. It was one of my only regrets during my degrading medical mystery. So, ashamed, despondent, and humiliated, back to my couch or bed I would collapse breathless and teary-eyed. I missed out on just about everything.

Every year I could expect to get the flu at minimum six times - chills, fever, all-over body aches - the works for three days at a time. If anyone near me had a sniffle, I too would succumb to a nasty cold. I had a difficult time standing and walking further than 100 or so feet at a time. Within a few steps I became weak, so exhausted I couldn't find the energy to lift my leg. I would get dizzy and feel extraordinarily weak - the way you feel when you have the flu and you can barely make it from the bed to the toilet. But for me, this was nearly every time I stood up. In public, I'd have to sit immediately to prevent passing out - I would descend upon rocks, sidewalks, and parking lot curbs; no place was safe and it was abundantly embarrassing. Even places like Costco and Walmart had nowhere to sit. I had to stop going. I always had my eye out for chairs, benches, ledges, really anything I could sit down on at a moment's notice.

In order to survive, I had to mourn so many losses of function and joy. I reluctantly and sadly gave up spin class, gym workouts, simple walks in nature, taking my children to the zoo or amusement parks, vacations that required standing, coaching soccer, skiing, time with friends, girl's weekends, traveling to see family, any semblance of a social life and anything that required me to be upright was off the table. Seriously, who is comfortable going to a party or a holiday and asking do you mind if I lie down on your couch instead of sitting here? I certainly wasn't so I remained very isolated in my home.

I could lie on a couch or a bed. I was that limited. I was alive but I certainly wasn't living. I started picking up groceries by ordering online and driving my car for personal delivery because I could no longer walk the length of a grocery store. I bought frozen meals I could easily heat up in the oven for my family because I could no longer stand long enough to chop vegetables and cook from scratch. Now a passion of mine, healthy eating for me and serving gorgeous meals to my family was buried too. I had to cut my work hours to the bare minimum so my family could survive but I could rest every other day and recover. I had to be seated at work at all times to try and disguise my illness. If a patient cancelled I would pass out on the treatment table until my receptionist woke me for the next person.

Low dose naltrexone was a medication I had researched on my own for years. I felt it was a drug worth trying. I begged for it. I presented studies and materials to any doctor I sought help from. But they just wouldn't listen to me. I knew anti-anxiety medications and antidepressants were the absolute wrong course of action for me personally but no doctor would listen to me. Once I said the words "But I can't get out of bed!" with tears brimming at my eyelids, I simply nailed my coffin shut. Once I had the misdiagnoses labeled on me no one could see past them. Having an electronic chart where every doctor could see the last one's misdiagnosis and misinterpretation of what I was relaying to them was keeping me trapped in misdiagnosis after misdiagnosis. Years went on like this. Those medications did zero for me except make me feel worse and cause inexplicable and enormous weight gain.

The medications failed me because I didn't have depression. The situation was undeniably depressing but this was not clinical depression. Instead, what they discovered may haunt you. I now realize my tearful pleading for a medical answer to my inextinguishable, unrelenting fatigue only further ignited their suspected diagnosis of anxiety and depression.

It took five years of asking for low dose naltrexone and not getting it, innumerable other horrendously failed treatments. The absolute worst treatment, by far was from a naturopath who put an IV of hydrochloric acid and ozone directly into my bloodstream. Immediate and debilitating, brutal side effects. My allopathic doctor said I could have without a doubt been killed. He made me swear I would never, ever do that treatment again. I had swallowed and shot myself with dozens of different types of drugs from different kinds of doctors from chiropractors to naturopaths to allergists to internists to endocrinologists and weight loss experts. All with failed drug regimens, therapies, and more drugs to finally convince a nurse practitioner to allow me to try this medication. At the time, I had the official diagnosis of myalgic encephalitis, hypothyroidism, PCOS with insulin-resistant metabolic syndrome, and the misdiagnosis of anxiety and depression. I ate like a bird and looked like… well, let's be compassionate here, I didn't look like I under-ate. All my doctors assumed I over-ate but I did not. No one seemed to believe me and they all commented on how I needed to lose weight. They blamed me for the side effects the drugs they wrongly prescribed were actually causing.

Low dose naltrexone was the catalyst that helped me get my life and health back. Although at the time, I didn't have the official diagnosis of Hashimoto's, only hypothyroidism, within weeks of being on low dose naltrexone my heart rate skyrocketed and my heart started to startlingly bang around inside my chest. I genuinely thought my heart was going to be bruised from hitting my ribcage so hard. I had read this happens with many Hashimoto's patients but I had never been diagnosed officially so I didn't think that would apply to me. My immune system was being modulated by low dose naltrexone and it was no longer attacking my thyroid. Therefore, I went rapidly from hypo to hyperthyroidism, and I no longer needed thyroid medication. I was originally told I would need thyroid medications for life. I made an emergency call to my nurse practitioner about my heart. She was very stern: I had to immediately stop all of my thyroid medications and I was never to return to them, ever.

Within months of being on low dose naltrexone, my pain eased and my POTS slowly started to get less intense. I was able to regain my ability to stand for longer periods of time. My pain level of 8 dropped to a pretty constant low level 3. I no longer get the flu. Rarely do I get a cold, maybe once a year.

The one year wait had finally come to an end and I got an appointment at Stanford Infectious Disease and The Mayo Clinic in Arizona. They confirmed my suspicion of dysautonomia with POTS. In addition, they diagnosed me with hEDS (hypermobile Ehlers-Danlos syndrome), Epstein-Barr virus, parvovirus, cytomegalovirus, walking pneumonia, a fungal infection in my blood and on my skin, a bacterial infection in my small intestine, Lyme disease, low vitamin D, and extremely low ferritin at level 9.

I did not have anxiety nor did I have depression - both brilliant doctors confirmed it. I was undoubtedly misdiagnosed over and over. Finally! I told all those doctors I was sick all of those years and goodness I was riddled with infections.

It took decades to be heard, seen, properly assessed, and diagnosed. In addition to my low dose naltrexone, I was prescribed several rounds of anti-fungal medications, nearly one year of multiple rounds of antibiotics that was $2,100 out of pocket for each ten day course (another story on that), years of antivirals, and finally, low dose naltrexone combined with low dose immune therapy for Lyme disease and weekly acupuncture for energy and pain relief. When I asked the doctors at Stanford University and Mayo Clinic if I should go off low dose naltrexone they said absolutely not.

I lost the majority of that pesky weight from those nasty medication side effects and now I teach others how to do the same. I am a fully upright, completely functioning, and an active person. I play tennis three times a week, cook healthy meals, paddleboard on the rivers and lakes, go out on date nights with my husband, organize social events for my friends and their husbands, and host every single holiday at my home with often a dozen guests. I continue to see patients while I stand and treat them. I offer telemedicine for medical mysteries and those suffering as I did. I am currently nearing the end of obtaining my doctorate in acupuncture and Chinese herbal medicine; the medicine I have been practicing locally and through telemedicine for nearly two and a half decades. I was able to spot an almost identical diagnosis in a colleague who lived out of state. I contacted her privately and told her I'm confident I may know what is wrong with her. I proceeded to tell her this is what you need to ask to get tested, this is what kind of provider you need and this is the medication you need to ask for. I saved her from the potential decades of despair. She reports she too is doing well. Do I need rest? Sometimes. Does my exhaustion flare here and there? Yes, it does. Can I manage it with a nap or resting for a day or two? Does acupuncture still enable me to do the work I was called to do? Absolutely.

This drug gave me my gorgeous, abundant, active, life back. Am I cured? There are no cures for most of those diseases I contracted while so very ill. Am I healthy? Yes! Am I grateful? Eternally.

Ellie, Australia – Multiple Autoimmune Conditions

I have suffered with multiple autoimmune diseases for my whole life. My hypothyroidism condition was getting worse, until I found a doctor who told me about LDN. I didn't know that desperate appointment I made would change my life. My hair has grown back, my eczema is at bay, and I no longer use thyroxine for my hypothyroidism. All my levels are normal. All thanks to LDN. It truly changed and saved my life.

Kerry, Canada - Hashimoto's, Fibromyalgia and Asthma

I was diagnosed with Hashimoto's thyroiditis at 15 years old, fibromyalgia in my 20s, and more recently, around the time I turned 40, diagnosed with adult-onset asthma. I have managed each of these conditions well with thyroid medication, diet, lifestyle, and traditional Chinese medicine, though some symptoms still remained. I decided to try LDN in hopes that it would decrease or eliminate these remaining symptoms. I also have a cancer risk gene mutation (Lynch syndrome), that significantly increases the risk of a number of cancers, and with the preliminary research on LDN suggesting an anti-cancer effect thought that that couldn't hurt either.

My low thyroid symptoms first began around 14 years old, and I got the official diagnosis of Hashimoto's thyroiditis at 15. I was not told it was Hashimoto's then, just hypothyroidism, and to take Synthroid for the rest of my life. My symptoms included being cold all the time, extreme fatigue, brain fog, and hair loss. Life was challenging until I got a diagnosis and treatment.

In my 20s I began having symptoms of non-exertion related muscle pain, muscle stiffness, chronic fatigue, and numbness and tingling in my arms and legs. My thyroid numbers looked ok and doctors ruled out MS. After a few years of these symptoms, I got the diagnosis of "fibromyalgia." Life was doable, but I was tired, sluggish, and always physically uncomfortable in my body. Some years into this I changed my diet dramatically, cutting out gluten, dairy, caffeine, alcohol, and sugar. This helped reduce a significant amount of the symptoms and I went on with life, despite daily muscle stiffness and pain (2-5/10). At one point I tried Lyrica for my fibro symptoms, which helped a lot, but it came with too many side effects and I didn't like that it was dangerous to come off of so I slowly stopped it.

The adult-onset asthma likely first began after a major pollution exposure to burning plastic in 2014 that left me with chronic bronchitis for a couple years, which eventually turned into asthma. I was prescribed Symbicort and a salbutamol puffer. I didn't like to take the Symbicort (steroid) so I rarely took that and just relied on my puffer as needed. With each winter though my asthma seemed to be getting worse, with my asthma triggers being cold, dry air and exertion.

I first heard of LDN in 2018 and wanted a family member to take it for their autoimmune condition but we couldn't find someone to prescribe it to them. I didn't even think about it for myself at the time. Last year, a dear friend mentioned that she had started LDN. This reminded me of the medication, and I began to look into it and consider it for myself. Researching through the LDN Research Trust website, I found my conditions were listed as "possibly helped" by LDN and I decided I wanted to try it. I mentioned it to my general practitioner (GP) and she said she had never heard of that use of naltrexone. I asked if I could send her some research on LDN and that if she felt it presented enough evidence, especially considering its good safety profile, to consider prescribing it to me. She agreed and, said she was willing to have a look. At our follow up appointment, she agreed to prescribe it to me. I have been with my GP for almost two decades, a long-standing relationship, and I feel this is why it was not a struggle to have her prescribe LDN. I feel if she didn't know me as well, she might not have been willing. I was the first of her patients, many years ago, to ask for desiccated thyroid; she had not heard of it when I asked and now she has many patients on it, so we had a history of exploring new-to-her medications together. Additionally, she knows that I have studied holistic nutrition, have a degree in biological science, and have a decent grasp of many biomedical concepts. At this same appointment I informed her that I would like to start at a dose of 0.5 mg LDN and aim to titrate up every two weeks by 0.5 mg, up to a max dose of 4.5 mg, depending on how I responded to it.

I started LDN in September 2022 on 0.5 mg/day at night. This resulted in insomnia for weeks that did not resolve. I experimented with going up in dose to 1 mg at night, thinking that perhaps it might help the insomnia, but it was just as bad at this dose. Seeking guidance from an LDN social media group support I switched to morning dosing which resolved the insomnia. Morning dosing also did not cause me any fatigue during the day. I attempted to titrate up to 1.5 mg/day morning dose but this brought back the insomnia, so I have remained at 1 mg/day morning dose until today. At this point this dose produces no side effects for me, while also results in multiple health benefits though I did have a few other side effects to start. The first was that it impacted my menstrual cycle, resulting in two shortened cycles, one of 15 days and one of 22, while my cycles were typically regular at 25 or 26 days. By the third cycle it was back to my norm. I also experienced an increase in hair loss when I first started LDN though this seems to have resolved. I can't say with certainty that either of these side effects were caused by LDN and not by something else, though the timing coincided with the start of the medication.

I noticed improvements in my mood within a few days of starting LDN. I had been feeling low in mood for some time after a series of challenging events, and LDN quickly improved this. Within a week or two my fibromyalgia pain and stiffness lessened. And within a couple months I noticed that I was not having asthma symptoms. It's hard to say how soon this occurred because my asthma was seasonal, and I started LDN during a time where my symptoms were minimal. By the time I would usually start using my puffer seasonally however, I just didn't need to, and amazingly, I have not used my puffer since before starting LDN.

I currently take thyroid hormone medications (Synthroid and desiccated thyroid), and LDN, and also take a lot of supplements.

Taking LDN has been a real boon to my health. I live in less pain and feel a stability in my health that I haven't felt for a very long time. I feel so grateful towards all the people who have advocated for the novel use of this drug. I think that LDN brings hope for so many who live with chronic illness and I feel excited to be a part of this movement.

Dorthe, Denmark - Multiple Autoimmune Conditions

I have had chronic pain in my jaw and pain in my knee for several years due to an injury. My life was horrible because of the constant pain. I was taking paracetamol 665 mg three times a day and diclofenac 40 mg three times a day. It helped my knee pain, not so much the jaw pain.

I attend a pain clinic in Denmark and 13 weeks ago they prescribed LDN for me. I started on 0.75 mg per day and increased the dose to 1.7 mg per day but every time I try to increase further I get terrible pain in my jaw. I've had a few nightmares and a bit of a headache but nothing else as side effects.

The first day on LDN I got a blast of energy and after a few days my sleep pattern changed for the better. I now sleep eight hours straight at night whereas I used to be up two or three times a night. My TSH is also going down. It's amazing.

I take other medications for Hashimoto's, IBS, eczema, ADHD and chronic stress. But LDN has made the most difference to my quality of life. It's been a life saver for me. I look better, feel better, sleep better – I would be terrified if I couldn't get it anymore because my quality of life would return to miserable, being in constant pain.

I am so grateful that I got the opportunity to try LDN. I hope that in time I can reduce my thyroid medications. I just feel so much better all round.

Joanna, Australia - Multiple Autoimmune Conditions

I was diagnosed with type 1 diabetes 35 years ago and had been struggling to manage blood sugars and high cholesterol. I have had numerous digestive disturbances (constipation, delayed gastric emptying, food allergies, bloating, etc.). I was diagnosed with CPTSD (complex post-traumatic stress disorder), and then later Hashimoto's, and it seemed every few years a new diagnosis. In addition to those already mentioned I've also been diagnosed with fibromyalgia, chronic painful skin rash, anxiety, transient depression, shifting joint pain, fatigue, adrenal exhaustion.

Over these past decades I just learned to tolerate the accumulating discomfort and tried my best to manage all the symptoms but it seriously affected my mental health because I could not participate in life fully. It was difficult to exercise without fear of the resulting severe pain, I was scared to eat because most things seemed to trigger some sort of negative reaction, despite following some of the most restrictive diets. It was difficult to maintain a job because of the fluctuating and random flare ups in mood, energy and inflammation.

My world was becoming smaller and smaller. I've invested tens of thousands of dollars on therapies and supplements to help me cope and alleviate the suffering over the years. My life was extremely difficult to navigate with so many autoimmune triggers. I'd confidently say that I've tried everything anyone could possibly think of - naturopaths, nutritionists, homeopaths, psychologists, endocrinologists, chiropractors, hypnotherapists, and numerous other specialist professionals. They were all helpful somewhat at delaying the momentum of autoimmune illness, but eventually I got to a point where nothing worked anymore. I felt hopeless and struggled to be optimistic about my future.

I've refused almost all doctors' recommendations to take cortisone, antidepressants, anxiolytics, cholesterol drugs and others because of my sensitivity to most drugs. I've managed to predominantly manage my symptoms with naturopathic supplements and by regularly seeing somatic practitioners to support my body coping with the stress of living with chronic illnesses. Prior to taking LDN the only prescription medications I have been on are insulin and thyroxine.

Obtaining a prescription for LDN was relatively easy for me because I had a very supportive integrative health practitioner, who suggested I try LDN but I hesitated because of my high reactivity to medications. I eventually looked it up online myself, prompted by an extreme flare-up which I could not manage with all my previous methods.

I only started on 1 mg of LDN four weeks ago. The effect was miraculous with the first dose. All my symptoms seemed to have disappeared overnight, I couldn't believe it. I was pain free, the joint pain disappeared, my throat no longer hurt, I could move with ease, and that was with my first dose. After one week my mood seemed to stabilize, I felt happier and my energy also regulated. The fatigue was gone and I felt like I had a new lease on life, it was truly remarkable! It has improved my sleep and I feel deeply rested in the morning, though not from first waking. Things improve within a short while, perhaps this is because I've slept so deeply. Shortly after this heavy feeling wears off I have really good energy for the entire day.

Two weeks into starting LDN I observed water retention, a heavy fullness in my body. It felt like I'd gained maybe 2-4 kg. I thought this was a side effect of LDN, but it appears that the water retention may likely be due to hormonal issues (and probably thyroid fluctuations) as I'm perimenopausal. It was probably the most severe case of water retention I'd had but considering there were a lot of adjustments being made in my body this month, I think maybe it was just part of the rebalancing process as the fluid retention has now completely gone. I've also noticed that perhaps my thyroxine will have to be reduced because in the last week or so my heart rate has episodically gone up and I feel breathless. I'm going for a follow up appointment next week so will be excited to see what my practitioner advises.

I'm not sure if 1 mg is my ideal dose because my practitioner advised that I increase it to 2 mg within the first month as I try to find the perfect dose.

I'm still taking insulin and will be monitoring my thyroid function to hopefully wean off the thyroxine, or try a natural bioidentical option to avoid the binders if necessary. I've also stopped seeing a therapist to help with fibromyalgia who I was seeing regularly for years, because I no longer have any muscle pain! I have reduced most of the supplements I was taking religiously to help me manage autoimmune symptoms as I'm feeling great and feel that I just don't need them any more – all this with just 1 mg naltrexone!

Taking LDN has been life saving for me. It's only been four weeks but I don't remember ever feeling this stable, happy and optimistic for my future and the possibility of healing from most of my accumulative health issues. I'm now exercising gently every day, am able to do house work, and many other activities I was previously unable to participate in. I feel I am also able to start letting go of the fear of food triggering an autoimmune response.

I feel grief for myself and many like me, who have unnecessarily suffered for many years because we were not informed about this miraculous drug. I feel like I have received the greatest gift, a second chance at life. I'm overwhelmed with gratitude for my integrative GP making this recommendation and thus changing the course of my destiny toward a now bright future.

Kimberely, US – Hashimoto's and Sjögren's Syndrome

Before I got sick, I was active and outdoors a lot. I was 39 when I noticed that that my mouth was dry and I had no idea why I suddenly seemed to have this problem – then it went on to dry eyes and nose, which was really uncomfortable. After several months the fatigue set in and I could barely get out of bed. I felt dreadful all the time, flu like symptoms, aches and pains. I tried all manner of medications, most giving me side effects that were worse than the original disease.

Eventually I went to a functional medicine doctor and wished I'd done so in the beginning. My doctor actually suggested LDN so I didn't have the problems that others have in getting it.

I had side effects with LDN initially, really problematic, but it was discovered that I was allergic to microcrystalline fillers – once I changed the filler to ginger root I was fine, no more side effects.

At around the third day I felt I had much more energy and was generally feeling much more optimistic about the future. At 2 months I was free of all aches and pains.

I did start to avoid gluten and dairy, and that perhaps helped some, but the LDN was the main thing. I went from a score of maybe 2 out of 10 to a happy 8 out of 10 on a quality-of-life scale in just 2 months. It was wonderful.

If I do flare, which is really occasional now, it isn't as debilitating as it used to be, I recover much quicker than before. I have to figure out what triggers my flares, something that I'm doing, or ingesting, is creating inflammation. It's obviously something I'm not doing all the time; I need to keep a food diary.

I am so grateful that I had a functional medicine doctor who thought outside the box and offered LDN to me, before that I hadn't heard of it. My life is back on track and I can now live again instead of existing.

My Hashimoto's antibody count had got as high as 13,000, which is horrifically high but since starting LDN the antibody figures are now 1,100 – which is still high but so much better than it was before, I'm expecting that to get better over time.

I've only been taking LDN for about 6 months. So now, the dry mouth, eyes and nose is better, not 100% but a good 90% - it's just a little irritating now. The fatigue and aches and pains are totally gone, I feel relatively normal now and sleep a lot better; feeling refreshed when I wake.

Jennifer, Australia – Mixed Connective Tissue Disease/Lupus

I first noticed symptoms in 2014 after I had Epstein-Barr virus. I became increasingly fatigued, my joints in my feet and ankles were increasingly painful and I started having headaches/migraines and brain fog, ulcerated tongue and palate and hair loss. I became increasingly unwell especially with fatigue, aching feet and nocturnal headaches. I couldn't function as a midwife and gradually decreased my shifts to barely part time. I saw numerous doctors and specialists whom thought it might be MS like my grandmother.

In November 2020 I couldn't get out of bed and I spent the next 18 months in bed due to bone crushing fatigue and pain. I have two teenage daughters who watched on in fear of me dying and my husband worked from home and moved his office into our bedroom to watch me. I was terribly ill.

My local rheumatologists would only give me hydroxychloroquine and prednisone, 35 mg per day, saying there is no such thing as seronegative lupus! My life was slipping away from me! I could rarely dress and feed myself. At times my daughters assisted me to shower and wash my hair. Morphine did not help the pain, codeine did help and ibuprofen was the most helpful with paracetamol regularly, however, I could not walk without a walking stick or aid.

Finally, I saw an immunologist in Sydney and commenced methotrexate 30 mg immediately with prednisone 35 mg and Plaquenil 400 mg. Over eight months I gradually decreased the prednisone and started to feel better. But the fatigue and joint pain continued, though I could walk a little further without aids. I tried mycophenolic acid for one month but the side effects were too difficult to manage. But I was feeling slightly better and ceased methotrexate after eight months especially after I had lost the bulk of my hair because of it. Fatigue and joint pain continued but were more bearable, though I could not work as the headaches and brain fog continued.

Before starting LDN I took prednisone 35 mg daily (now only 8 mg daily), hydroxychloroquine 400 mg daily, methotrexate 30 mg weekly for eight months, which caused terrible hair loss, mycophenolic acid for one month, aspirin 50 mg daily, fish oil daily, CoQ10 daily, Chinese herbs from a Chinese acupuncturist/herbalist, reishi and lions mane tinctures.

I heard about LDN on a lupus support group online and I then started researching it. I then borrowed *The LDN Book, Volume 2* from our local library. Then I purchased the book as I thought it was so great and I wanted to lend it to my friends whom I thought could benefit from LDN. I have also lent the book to my GP practice for the other GPs to read it, as I think LDN is such an important drug for so many people.

I was so lucky that my GP had just watched a video about LDN on YouTube the previous week and was open to prescribing it. I started LDN in July 2022 at 1.5 mg for a few months. I increased to 3 mg for another three months and then went up to 4.5 mg daily, which is the dose that works well for me now.

I had moderately strong headaches for the first three days but they were easily relieved with paracetamol. By day five the headaches had completely cleared and I had no other negative side effects at all.

By the end of the first week, I noticed my fatigue was lifting for the first time in nine years!!!

I still take four prescription medications and six non-prescription supplements but the major changes came after that first week on LDN. I now have energy and can think clearly! Most importantly I am able to return to work after two years of being bed ridden! I believe this is a great drug and I tell as many people as possible about it. It has changed my life for the better.

Also, my daughter has a lot of lupus symptoms, especially brain fog and fatigue. Our GP started her on LDN and she feels so much better on it! She reports that her brain fog has lifted completely and she's doing much better at school which is wonderful, especially as this is her final year, and she starts trial HSC exams next week. Her academic marks are now exceptional and she usually gets 19/20 for most exams and assignments.

My brother, who has suffered major depression and PTSD, started LDN last year, with my encouragement, and he now reports that he feels so much better and is now looking forward in his life and feels that finally his depression has lifted.

I think LDN should be routinely given to any person with an autoimmune disease. Secondly, it should be routinely given to any child with a behavioural issue as there is evidence for it helping there too.

Kimberly, USA - Sjögren's Syndrome and Hashimoto's

My health problems began around 2008 when I was diagnosed with oral cancer on my tongue after I had been complaining of extreme dry mouth beforehand. In August 2021 I was diagnosed with Sjögren's syndrome which had made itself more evident after having the COVID virus multiple times. Hashimoto's was diagnosed around the same time through blood work.

At the first onset of symptoms and the oral cancer, I had five different surgeries to remove cancer from my tongue but we didn't know what the cause was at the time. Fast forward to 2021, when I started having all the other symptoms such as terrible joint and muscle pain, debilitating fatigue, extreme dry eyes, dry nose, dry mouth, and all kinds of gastrointestinal issues. I actually had to take some medical leave for several months from my job at the time and I ended up getting laid off shortly thereafter.

It completely changed my life because I was unable to do the things I once could do. I wasn't even able to do my computer desk job for a full day, I wasn't able to take my dogs for walks. I was barely able to do any kind of housework, and I didn't have any energy or the ability to do anything fun. I could no longer do hiking and I could no longer do CrossFit which I loved, and going to festivals and things like that were out of the question. Everything became something I was unable to do.

I was started on hydroxychloroquine for a while and it did seem to help the joint pain but not so much the fatigue. After a while I noticed that hydroxychloroquine had started giving me heart issues. After everything else was ruled out through extensive cardiac testing, I just decided to stop taking hydroxychloroquine and sure enough my heart symptoms went away.

I had tried meloxicam as well for the pain and it helped a lot but it's very toxic as well and can cause much havoc on your stomach and other organs. I stopped that pretty quickly too. I tried to do some physical therapy but it was just too much at the time and I was unable to do it without going into a full autoimmune flare.

I was also trying over-the-counter herbal supplements such as turmeric and vitamin B, which I still take because they're very beneficial, but they just weren't giving me the relief I really wanted.

I had actually heard about LDN from an acquaintance on social media when I was first diagnosed, but then I didn't do much research on it and since none of my doctors mentioned it, I kind of forgot about it. I did finally get a prescription for it when I told my functional medicine doctor that despite what I was taking and trying to do, I was still having joint and muscle pain and still having tons of fatigue that interfered with my daily life. So it was September 2022 when I finally got a prescription for LDN, two years after my initial diagnoses.

I started on 1.5 mg of LDN and increased the dose until I settled on my ideal dose of 4.5 mg every morning and 1.5 mg in the afternoon. This works well for me. I did initially have a reaction to the Avicel (microcrystalline cellulose) but once I'd figured that out and switched to ginger root as a filler I had no further issues.

There were a couple of occasions where I tried to titrate up too quickly and I had a bit of a headache and maybe a little bit of anxiety but they went away quickly. I also noticed I was unable to take the dosing at night time because I would wake up around 3 or 4 a.m. wide awake and unable to fall back to sleep and that didn't work for my personal schedule. I would say it caused some insomnia with nighttime dosing which is why I switched to daytime dosing. Once I'd found my ideal filler, time and dose I had no further issues with negative side effects.

I noticed better sleep within a couple of days of starting LDN and even some relief from the joint pain. Within three weeks I noticed full benefit with the joint pain and muscle pain relief, as well as the fatigue relief around seven months, after I found my dose that works for me.

The only prescribed medications I take now are lisinopril for high blood pressure, which I don't even believe I need anymore, and the LDN.

Taking LDN means I can have a very large portion of my prior life back! I can actually function like a normal adult and do the things that I need to get done and also have energy left over to do the fun things that I enjoy.

LDN is a game changer for me and I am so thankful that I was able to get it and have it work for me. I would have probably had to quit my job and been put on disability if I hadn't found it when I did. It is truly a lifesaver!

Paul, Canada – Chronic Pain, Cancer, Arthritis and TMJ

I'm 66 years old now, I've had TMJ for 30-years, there doesn't seem to be a solution to TMJ in the allopathic world. Chronic pain has destroyed my sleep which makes things worse, that all started about 25-years ago – it was really hard to get comfortable and I was exhausted. The chronic pain was pretty much everywhere, shoulders, neck, legs, back and my hips were really bad. My doctor calls this arthritis but given its sudden start I suspect some medication I was on for a prostrate problem – I was fine before taking those, apart from the TMJ of course, that had got worse. Pain relief was Valium, NSAIDs, meloxicam and more on top of those because they really weren't touching the pain – the pain was so bad I just sat and cried, it was a hopeless situation.

I did see a pain specialist, which was pretty much the same old stuff, more drugs – I refused morphine – I didn't want that, I've seen the misery that can cause first hand with a friend of mine. I was just miserable. It was a horrible existence.

There didn't seem to be a solution anywhere – just symptom control – that didn't work, but did give side effects that were unpleasant and I was already in a bad place.

I was diagnosed with prostate cancer too – I was given Anandron which has many permanent side effects so I didn't want to be on that too long.

Last year I heard about LDN, I read a lot of research papers on it and the fact that my regular doctors hadn't suggested it – because it wasn't "Standard Care" - I thought was intriguing. It seemed like LDN could help all of my ailments – and of course I could afford it – unlike the other treatments I'd been offered.

I started LDN at 1.5 mg and increased every week by 1 mg until I got to 4.5 mg. The very first night of taking LDN I slept five hours solid, that was wonderful. I started with the vivid dreams toward the end of the first week but I actually enjoyed those – I looked forward to the dreams, though that stopped after the first month. The very first time I slept a full 8 hours was in the first month, that was amazing. I started to realise, toward the end of the second month, that I had much better movement, my knees and hips were "looser" and didn't hurt so bad. By the end of month 3 my pain was so much less that I didn't need the pain killers at bedtime, I was in a constant state of amazement for quite a while that my quality of life had improved so much.

It is disappointing, and saddening, that our health care system won't even consider LDN as a first line treatment for so many immune system issues. My family doctor isn't impressed at all with my choice to refuse his drugs and take one that I had sourced myself – he seems to think is a narcotic for some reason, I don't understand how they can be so confident about their negative statements when they are so wrong.

My prostate cancer hasn't really progressed, the tests aren't showing that anything there is worse but hopefully when I next have a check up it will show that it is getting less and less. I stopped taking the Anandron before I started the LDN.

I'm happy now that I can enjoy my life without the pain – even the TMJ pain is more of an irritation now than a debilitating sleep destroyer – I'm really happy with that.

Deborah, USA – Multiple Autoimmune Conditions

My osteoarthritis started giving me more trouble in 2020, overwhelming my ability to cope with what had been decades-long chronic pain. I was diagnosed in March 2021 with Ehlers-Danlos syndrome (EDS). In 2022 I finally got a diagnosis for small fiber neuropathy (SFN) which I'd had since 1980 but no doctor seemed able to tell me what it was.

I have Crohn's disease, for which I'm taking balsalazide. I take a muscle relaxant called cyclobenzaprine and I take trazodone at night though even with that it was hard to sleep.

For the osteoarthritis I was given Celebrex, gabapentin for the SFN and nothing for the EDS. These drugs were helpful but not helpful enough to give me a reasonable day.

I have gained quite a bit of weight but it's really hard to say whether that's my thyroid that I'm having issues with or gabapentin which caused weight gain when I started it. I have no idea. But I will see my endocrinologist in a month and we'll figure out what's going on hopefully. I was taking Tapazole for the Graves' disease until last December – I may have to go back on that.

The small fiber neuropathy affects many things beside the sensations in my hands and feet and one thing I think it was affecting was my hearing, particularly in my right ear.

I had been on various social media groups dedicated to these ailments for a few years and I had seen mention of LDN on the EDS group. I didn't think I was "bad enough" to try something new for a long time but then realized I could actually be better than I was, if LDN were to work. So last year, around February 2022, I took the leap and found an online option that provided a physician to prescribe it. From the very first dose I felt somewhat better!

I started at 1.5 mg and titrated up 1.5 every few weeks. Initially I had trouble getting to sleep, but that wasn't unusual for me. I persevered for around three or four months but then I moved to taking it in the morning and the sleep issues went away.

I wanted to see whether I could get more out of LDN so I experimented for a few days going up to 6 mg and that was really helpful, it was great, my right ear issues went away and now my hearing is much better. Then, when we moved in November, I felt really crap so I went up to 7.5 and again it really helped a lot. I've been on 7.5 for about eight weeks and feel a lot less crap.

Apart from sleeplessness, which I had anyway – maybe LDN made that worse, maybe not, but I had no other negative side effects. Going from 3 mg to 4.5 mg I had like a blissful experience, but I was also extremely overwhelmed by visual stimuli which made me nauseous. I was so happy having this really positive emotional experience and then after one or two doses that feeling went away and I was just a lot better all round.

The benefits are huge. Even though I take all this other medication and feel crap on it, the benefits of LDN are still huge. I have more energy, I'm much less limited. My widespread muscular pain has been much better. The gabapentin helped but hadn't eliminated the pain. That was so much better when taking LDN. I have mainly focal pain now, some in my neck and my back. I feel that my moods are so much better and more stable, I feel more solid inside, I don't have all those ups and downs anymore.

I'm now sleeping deeper than I've slept in decades. I had a brain injury in 1992 and had a real struggle getting to sleep but now it's so much better on LDN. Cognitive clarity is so much better – the brain fog has gone and LDN is the only thing that has positively impacted my brain fog. I used to have only an hour or two of mental clarity now I can read again because I can concentrate better and have many more hours of clarity a day.

I now have very low symptom activity with the Crohn's disease since being on LDN. I'm having less temperature dysregulation since LDN. I used to be freezing cold then steaming hot but that is much better now.

LDN has been an enormous help to me with pain (neuropathic, muscular, joint), mood, cognitive abilities, and energy. I am very fortunate that it started helping with the first dose. It's been the only thing I've done that significantly reduced mental fog, and increased sensation in my hands and feet. It was vital to helping us move house recently. I don't know how I would have accomplished that without LDN. It makes a real difference every day.

Sita Huber, BHSc (Nutritional Medicine), Canada - POTS/hEDS/MCAS

I have always described my health as "high maintenance". I was teased by health and fitness colleagues for my resorting to "air weights"- for some reason I knew I had to work hard on my health, and that I fell apart more easily than others. I completed a health science degree in nutritional medicine in Australia in 2008, in an effort to understand the role of nutrition in my health, and it opened up a whole world of lifestyle medicine.

While many things such as acupuncture, Pilates, mindfulness, supplements and a gluten-free low-carb diet helped me over the years, I have been on a health roller coaster my whole life with diagnoses of IBS (2008), joint hypermobility (2012) and chronic pain for seven years, as well as a history of what we would call high-functioning anxiety.

In 2018 I moved back to Canada from Australia and the stress of a family emergency triggered a decline in my health. High stress has always crippled me, even though I feel mentally strong and utilize many methods of self-care including daily meditation since 2014.

I finally heard about POTS and it fit my symptoms. I was diagnosed in Feb 2021, after at least two years of feeling unable to be myself, severe insomnia, "panic" attacks, burning feet, internal tremors, dizziness, severe tachycardia, post-exercise fatigue and exhaustion. Prior to the POTS diagnosis I had a neurofeedback brain scan and it showed high amygdala activity - in line with PTSD - so I started direct neurofeedback sessions and EMDR – thinking I had PTSD.

By my own research I eventually came across information about EDS and am now finally diagnosed with hEDS with POTS. Along with this I show symptoms of MCAS and understand this to be a common "trifecta".

For treatment of POTS I applied my typical "A" student approach and learned and tried everything. My cardiologist only had to approve, as everything I was doing (recumbent exercise/aggressive hydration/ medications/compression) was helping with the tachycardia side of POTS.

Even with all this effort I still didn't feel right and was living as a fragment of my previous self, unable to handle travel, exhausted after grocery shopping or climbing stairs. I described every day as walking a thin line on a cliff edge not knowing when a wind would come and blow me over. The crashes were hard.

Through my own research (again) I asked my GP to start histamine therapy. This made an incredible and surprising difference and I started to sleep better. The hotness in my feet eased.

Last summer (2022) I watched all of the dysautonomia international conference lectures and came across one on LDN. I asked my GP if I could try this in October and she was familiar enough with it to prescribe it. I have worked with her on dosing, based on information I got from the LDN Research Trust. I also had to switch the filler as the Avicel gave me severe upper abdominal pain.

In the first week I started LDN I was able to attend an in-store event for my job. It was such a surprise. I didn't feel exhausted, I didn't crash after. That was on 0.5 mg.

I titrated by 0.5 mg every two weeks since then, up to 5.5 mg and eventually came to twice a day dosing based on a new study from the Netherlands about cytokine activity. Currently, because of LDN I am able to function like a normal person.

I credit LDN for giving me my life back. I can be creative in my job again, I can write, I can talk and finish sentences without being exhausted. I sleep well! I have less pain and internal distress. I can exercise an hour a day if I want to. I am so grateful for what LDN has done for me. I can't believe it wasn't on my radar before 2022.

My wish now is that more people with EDS, POTS and other autoimmune, autoinflammatory or chronic conditions can be offered LDN sooner rather than later. I feel like I lost a chunk of my life that I can never get back. Imagine if I'd have found LDN 15 years ago when I had so much daily pain? I love the way I feel on LDN and have nothing negative to say about it whatsoever. LDN is a true gift. A miracle. The closest thing I've ever found to a cure for my "incurable" conditions.

Sherri, USA – Small Fiber Neuropathy and Sjögren's Syndrome

I was diagnosed with small fiber neuropathy (SFN) at Johns Hopkins in Baltimore. I already had Sjögren's syndrome. The very knowledgeable rheumatologist/neurologist prescribed Plaquenil, however, I told him I was going to try LDN first. I did and I got my life back. I went from crying in bed, all day in pain, to walking 15 miles per week and living my best life. I've been taking LDN for six years. And they say I'm aging backwards! LDN is a lifesaver.

Bridget, USA - Sjögren's and Epstein-Barr Virus

My health problems started sometime after having my triplets in the fall of 2009. The first thing I noticed was fatigue. I wrote it off for a while, because you're supposed to be tired when raising triplets, right? Unfortunately, I went from "tired" to almost unable to get off the couch, let alone walk up the stairs of my two story house.

I made an appointment with my family's naturopath, and she diagnosed me with adrenal fatigue. After a few weeks of using her protocol, I was functional again. Not great, but at least it was an improvement. Things remained fairly stable until 2012, when seemingly out of nowhere, I got strange sores on my skin. I went to my primary doctor who gave me antibiotics and referred me to a dermatologist. Over the years, I saw three different dermatologists, and none were helpful. One even suggested that my issues were self inflicted.

The constant antibiotics were making me sicker, and I was no closer to a diagnosis. By 2018, not only was my skin condition horrendous, but my fatigue was back, and I began suffering from a lot of joint pain. At some point I developed chronic dry eye, and chronic sore throat as well. I didn't pay much attention to those, because I could push through it. The other symptoms, however, drove me to seek out a Lyme specialist. It was at this time, about eight years after my symptoms began, that I was diagnosed with Sjögren's, Epstein-Barr virus, B12 deficiency, and borderline anemia. Somehow, no other doctor had ever ordered blood work for these things.

I was beyond relieved to have an actual, provable diagnosis that explained at least some of my ailments. Unfortunately, the treatment the Lyme doctor put me on was extremely expensive, and didn't help much. In 2020, I stopped seeing her, and went to a rheumatologist. I was offered hydroxychloroquine, but refused due to the chance of permanent retinal damage. I will add here that at some point, I don't remember exactly when, I was diagnosed with discoid lupus, by my symptoms only, as no one would agree to do a biopsy because it leaves a noticeable scar. After refusing HCQ, I thought I would have to live with these illnesses forever. Unfortunately, things continued to get worse. By 2022, I was experiencing symptoms of interstitial cystitis, and mast cell activation syndrome.

Every day was a struggle, and I was not enjoying being alive. My symptoms, prior to LDN, were as follows: joint pain, muscle pain, fatigue, brain fog, skin lesions, dry eye, dry sore throat, painful bladder, frequent urination, chronic hives. I was also having some issues with my eyesight, and oral health, no doubt due to my Sjögren's disease.

I found out about LDN in the summer of 2022, in a Sjögren's support group on social media. By fall of 2022, I was prescribed a starting dose of 1.5 mg, with instructions to move up to 4.5 within 20 days. The first three days I experienced insomnia, dizziness, and vivid dreams. After that, the only side effect that remained is vivid dreams. As for the benefits, within two weeks, my joint and muscle pain greatly decreased, and my energy levels improved dramatically. Within a few months, I noticed improvements in every one of my symptoms. My joint and bladder pains are completely gone, and I almost never get hives anymore.

My mind is sharp again, and I have enough energy to get through the day. My eyesight improved, and this was confirmed by my ophthalmologist. My dental health improved as well. I rarely get discoid lesions anymore, and when I do, they heal much more quickly. I still deal with dry eyes and throat, but not as severe as it was. Now, at 40 years old, I feel better than I have in 13 years. LDN gave me my life back.

Patti, USA – Multiple Autoimmune Conditions

I take LDN for autonomic small fiber neuropathy and ME/CFS that I developed after a missed diagnosis of Guillain-Barré in 2018. Since 2018 I have had post-exertion malaise, fatigue, brain fog, cardiac arrhythmias, severe muscle cramping in my feet and legs, severe shortness of breath even with daily activities. Living life was very hard. I even lost my job. The fatigue was the worst. It felt like all the ATP in my mitochondria was depleted.

I found taking NAC, glutamine and glutathione helped the fatigue the most. An essential oil roll-on for pain helped the most with the unpredictable muscle cramps that felt like I was being electrocuted. Magnesium did nothing for the cramping.

One of the cardiac arrhythmias is atrial fibrillation which caused my left atrium to enlarge to the point it was pushing the septum into the right atrium. I also started Eliquis, an anticoagulant.

My naturopathic doctor suggested LDN in 2022. I started at 0.5 mg slowly increasing to 5 mg. At 2.5 mg orally I experienced nausea and a dull headache. When I switched to sublingual I have been able to consistently tolerate 5 mg with no side effects.

Taking LDN has improved the quality of my life significantly! I have more energy, the brain fog is MUCH better, the different arrhythmias are rare if not gone, I still have dyspnea on exertion but it is not as severe.

I recently had surgery and had to stop the LDN. That is when I realized just how much the LDN has helped me to feel better. I am so happy to be taking it once again.

I haven't had to take the NAC, glutamine, and glutathione. The muscle cramping is virtually non-existent. I would say that LDN has virtually saved both my sanity and my life!

Cheryl, USA – CRPS and EDS

My daughter was dealing with unbearable pain from complex regional pain syndrome and undiagnosed hypermobile Ehlers-Danlos syndrome. Combining gabapentin with low dose naltrexone put my daughter's severe neuropathic pain in remission. It was prescribed in 2014 and took a few months to get its full effect.

My daughter had to start at a low dose and go up incrementally. She was sleeping better and her mood improved as the unbearable pain and allodynia she was coping with decreased as she used LDN. After six months on it, she had what we call a two week "fizzle period" where she had a bad migraine, a pain flare … and then the neuropathic pain went into full remission.

The pain has only returned during periods of severe stress or when she tried to decrease her gabapentin or stop her LDN for surgery.

LDN has been a miracle drug for her CRPS and we are so thankful her pain doctor had researched it and was willing to prescribe it for her. It has saved her life.

Elizabeth, USA – Multiple Autoimmune Conditions

I currently take naltrexone 4 mg in the morning and 5 mg in the evening. I started taking it six to eight months ago. I use it for a few different conditions: fibromyalgia, chronic pain, CIRS (chronic inflammatory response syndrome), migraines, SIBO, Raynaud's phenomenon, PTSD, brain fog, histamine intolerance, etc., etc., etc.

My health began to spiral around 12 years ago. I had strange neurological symptoms, pain, breathing troubles, hair loss, degeneration of my spine, rashes, upper respiratory infections. I even had C. diff. My husband and I were terrified. We had a young child and I could hardly care for him.

I saw many specialists and they'd tell me that they couldn't really tell me what was wrong and they tried to treat all of the above symptoms separately. One doctor thought I had MS. Another thought it was psychosomatic. I felt hopeless until I took a leap of faith with another specialist that diagnosed CIRS, which is similar to Lyme disease. It's a horrible systemic inflammation that cascades throughout your body causing problems with your brain, all organs, joints, etc. In fact, almost all of my symptoms stem from this illness but it's complicated by my fibrosis in my lungs, degenerative spine issues and now, an enlarged pulmonary artery.

My entire life, I was always so incredibly healthy, athletic and fit until suddenly, I was not. And everything sort of started happening at once. Scary stuff.

Fast forward to now. Recently I read online about LDN. It was hard to believe that a medication, taken in tiny amounts, could treat all the conditions that were listed on the LDN Research Trust website. I listened to interviews, watched YouTube testimonials, bought the three books and immersed myself in learning. I asked my doctor about it and she knew about it, wrote the prescription for me and my journey began.

We slowly titrated up to my current dose (9 mg split between a.m. and p.m.). I don't recall experiencing any side effects. I just remember going into the kitchen one morning and seeing the look of shock on my husband's face. He said, "You're upright. You walked in here like normal!" I hadn't done that in so long. It hurt to get out of bed. I was often hunched over, limping, in excruciating pain. This just kept getting better.

I started doing Pilates twice a week, walking, and interacting with people. I smiled. A lot. My husband even told me that I am nicer! LDN has really taken the edge off this pain, given me a bit of my life back. I'm just beginning my journey but I'm telling everyone who has noticed and anyone who'll listen, that this medication, in small doses, can be incredibly life changing.

In fact, I had my 80-year-old mother start taking it and it's made her so much younger and active. She also has CIRS and possibly fibromyalgia. I asked her if she had noticed a change. She said that this has absolutely made a profound difference in her ability to function in her daily life. The aches, the pains, etc. have all been ratcheted down many notches. I'm so happy about this.

I still take 53 pills a day (both prescription and supplements) but am slowly knocking meds off my list each few months. My doctor has really been impressed with this and is going to speak to her many Lyme and CIRS patients about this. I even offered to chat with them if they wanted.

Thank you for bringing this to the people that need it and I am here as an example of how truly life changing it can be. Taking LDN is a gift to me; I feel like it's pushing pause on many of my debilitating symptoms so I can get more out of my life, to live with my family and just be in an all-around better place, both physically and mentally.

Julia, USA – Multiple Autoimmune Conditions

I first noticed symptoms in January 2020. My life became very difficult with chronic pain, mainly in my joints but also in muscles and tendons. I had severe B12 deficiency so was treated with frequent B12 injections. I was offered many mainstream drugs for the unspecified autoimmune arthritis (as per my rheumatologist, though I did test above range for RA), but I resisted trying all but meloxicam, but I have stomach issues from the pernicious anemia so I couldn't take that often. I eventually agreed to take hydroxychloroquine which landed me in the ER. I just couldn't tolerate it and I didn't want biologics either so I researched and found LDN.

I found people talking about LDN on a social media group for autoimmune diseases. It really piqued my interest due to the low side effects and the great results other people were having with it. I used an online prescriber to get my prescription, which luckily wasn't too difficult. So in December 2022 I started LDN on 1.5 mg per day and increased up to 3 mg which is my best dose.

I did initially have side effects, just a couple of months of sleep disturbance which wore off. Other than that I had no other adverse effects at all.

About three weeks in I noticed decreased muscle, joint and tendon pain and this has continued to present. I only take LDN now and it has given me my life back! I was miserable and terrified that biologics would be my only option and the only next step. I really didn't want those.

I am so thankful that I found LDN. I tell everyone and anyone who needs help with autoimmune diseases about it. It could help so many people if only it were offered as a first line treatment.

Elaine, UK – Multiple Autoimmune Conditions

Since 1983 my life has been totally ruined by my conditions. I cannot work and up until a few years ago, was totally bedbound.

I think I tried every "miracle cure" and new drug going over the last 40 years. Nothing worked. I was offered painkillers, injections into my joints, surgery, radioactive x-rays and creams. Nothing worked.

You name it, I've tried it. I was on a high dose of opioid medications that weren't working before I went to a private rheumatologist and was prescribed LDN. This was in June 2021.

Getting the prescription was easy, getting it filled was impossible in Wales. My husband paid almost £500 for a supply of capsules from a local pharmacy. These made me very ill due to me reacting to the Avicel filler which we eventually had changed to something I could tolerate.

I started on 3 mg, but it was way too high so I stopped and restarted at 0.5 mg and worked my way up to what I now consider to be my perfect dose of 15 mg per day.

The only side effect from the LDN I have experienced is vivid dreams but these only lasted two weeks and then went away. I no longer suffer any negative side effects to LDN.

At 12 to 13 months I noticed I was in less pain, was more awake and my brain fog had disappeared.

I still take levothyroxine, fexofenadine and venlafaxine. I was on 35 tablets a day before I started LDN, now I take just these three.

Taking LDN means the difference from being totally bedbound and feeling very ill to being able to spend time downstairs with my husband and being able to do things around the house. It's changed my life for the better. I'm no longer bedbound and I'm able to do things I haven't been able to do in donkey's years. I have no brain fog, far less pain and am awake and alert for longer periods every day. LDN has changed my life for the better.

Sharol, USA – Fibromyalgia and Rheumatoid Arthritis

I started taking LDN for fibromyalgia pain and to try and rid my lower legs of tactile allodynia. I have had fibromyalgia and RA since I was nine years old, I am now 51. I was not diagnosed until age 28 with fibromyalgia.

Living with chronic pain is terrible, it can make you so depressed. The main symptom of my fibromyalgia was back pain, especially in the winter. I have tried so many different medications to try to alleviate the pain. I have tried muscle relaxers such as Flexeril, other medications such as Trazadone, gabapentin, Lyrica, Cymbalta, and I was even on narcotics.

At first I was on Lortab and soon that stopped working so I was put on Percocet. I hated being on narcotics due to the way it made me feel plus it never really took away the pain.

In January 2019 my rheumatologist prescribed LDN. I approached her with the idea and she said it was for alcoholism and narcotic abuse users. I explained to her in great detail what LDN is good for and the benefits and explained the dosing as well to her. She was very receptive and was willing to give it a try for my fibro pain. I told her how I would like to start at 0.5 mg and increase by 0.5 mg every month.

I started taking LDN in the mornings as I was afraid of increased insomnia. After one week the pain in my back and knees were terribly worse. That only lasted roughly five to seven days and I was feeling so much better after ten days.

By month two I was on 1 mg and asked the doctor to increase me every two weeks until I reached 3 mg which did happen. By the end of the third month, I was on 3 mg and started to feel great. The pain in my back was not as bad at all. I stayed on 3 mg for about eight months and noticed some break-through pain so I increased to 4 mg. I have been on 4 mg now for over two years and I have zero pain in my back. It has been so amazing. I no longer have to take any form of a narcotic ever since starting on LDN and finding my "sweet spot." I currently take six medications, none relating to fibromyalgia though.

One other positive that has come from taking LDN is that after 13 years with chronic kidney stones I no longer have any kidney stones! I attribute this totally to taking LDN. I am on medication as well for them but all the years prior to the last two years I usually have two to five stones in each kidney on my yearly exam and for the past two years I have not had one. I am hoping to get rid of that medication and see if the stones don't come back due to being on LDN.

I didn't really think that LDN had helped my tactile allodynia much, but when I take a break from taking LDN I can tell it has helped some for that pain in my lower legs.

Initially I started taking it in the morning due to being afraid that it would make my insomnia worse. Two months into taking LDN I had to switch to nights due to having to take a nap in the afternoons because I was extremely tired and couldn't stay awake. Now that I am taking it right before bed it has actually helped with my insomnia.

Deena, USA - Undifferentiated Connective Tissue Disease

I started taking LDN two years ago and my autoimmune issues became 75-90% resolved.

When I was 28 years old, I woke up one morning unable to walk because my ankles were so swollen and stiff. I felt excruciating pain. My doctor determined from my symptoms, family history and the blood test result that I had rheumatoid arthritis. She predicted that I would be unable to walk and that I would be using a wheel chair in a few years.

In the months that followed I was in and out of her office and being referred to specialists for chronic infections and migrating arthritic pain as well as hives and rash from sun exposure.

One day after my blood work she entered the exam room, crouched below me on one knee as I sat waiting for my latest blood test results. I was stunned as she started slowly to explain that my blood results were indicating something far more serious that RA. She then explained I had lupus. She explained how I could have sudden organ failure and possibly die.

When I saw the specialist, she confirmed I had lupus. She began writing two prescriptions. One was a chemotherapy drug and the other an anti-malarial drug. I asked her to stop writing and tell me if the drugs would prevent kidney failure. At the lupus support meetings I had been attending I heard women say that they went to bed feeling okay and woke up in the middle of the night so ill they had to be rushed to the hospital where it was determined they had kidney failure. She paused a moment and looked at me thoughtfully and she then replied that she couldn't guarantee it wouldn't happen. I decided not to take the medications.

The symptoms were extreme itchiness and infections from less than a few minutes of UV exposure from the sun, chronic fatigue that kept me bedridden feeling like I'd been hit by a truck, chronic HSV-2/shingles; chronic joint, nerve, muscle, and bone pain; chemical sensitivity, IBS, GERD, intense sciatica pain, vulvodynia, carpal tunnel pain so intense I had to have surgery and the surgeon told me he'd never seen pressure on the nerves to that degree, histamine intolerance with food as well as extreme reactions to bug bites; vestibular migraine which manifested with extreme vertigo, violent vomiting, and diarrhea, insomnia, depression, anxiety, panic attacks, neurological symptoms that I experienced as recurrent night terrors. I was temporarily paralyzed upon waking one time and I even had a brief episode of dementia on another occasion. I have a drawer full of different braces for fingers, wrists, back, ankles and knees.

My doctor, who has lupus, changed my diagnosis to undifferentiated connective tissue disease (UCTD) because I have not had organ failure.

If only I'd been offered LDN sooner. I now sleep deep and feel happy since taking LDN. Eating an anti-inflammatory diet helped somewhat in the past but in combination with taking LDN I am healthier than I've been in 40 years. I am grateful to the LDN Research Trust and hope my story helps someone.

Julie, USA – Multiple Autoimmune Conditions

I was diagnosed with breast cancer in 2006 and had a left mastectomy and chemotherapy.

Then in 2022 I was diagnosed with breast cancer in my right breast and had a lumpectomy and radiation. Six years ago I was diagnosed with hypothyroidism and five years ago was diagnosed with diverticulitis.

I'm on medication for all of these but I did get off of 1 mg of Klonopin after ten years. I took that for anxiety and insomnia. That's a huge thing to not be on a benzodiazepine.

I started LDN approximately six years ago on 4.5 mg. From the beginning of the first week the side effects were a little bit of a headache and insomnia for about seven to ten days and then that passed.

I have been missing a week every now and then as it cost me almost $50 a month in the compound pharmacy but I have been as consistent as I can on LDN to manage pain. The pain that I have is nothing compared to when I am not on LDN. I do notice inflammation and the arthritis is still there of course but not as bad so I'm able to last at least until maybe 3 or 4 o'clock before having to lay down and rest whereas prior to LDN I was tired most of the time.

One of the most positive side effects from the LDN was that I no longer had cravings for alcohol because I was a social drinker, plus beer and wine at night after work often and I was also a stress drinker. Before LDN I wanted to have a couple beers or a couple glasses of wine and now I have no desire and usually pour out the glass because I have no desire for more.

I'm very grateful to say five years on LDN 4.5 mg helps with my pain, breast cancer twice and many surgeries. I consider that the most fantastic side effect, that I was not looking for, was no cravings for alcohol which is a big bonus for me.

Michael, USA – Neuropathy and Arthritis

About eight years ago, I was diagnosed with idiopathic neuropathy as well as arthritis in my feet and back. It seems like a lot of bad things started happening to my body all at once and I suddenly felt out of control. I had always been a worldwide adventurer and my job required a lot of air travel and hotel stays. Suddenly, I was applying for disability and on the sofa. I took an early retirement, got on disability, and no longer recognized myself.

My journey toward healing included trips to multiple neurologists, a trip to the Mayo Clinic, visits with rheumatologists, pain doctors, orthopedists, physiatrists, and many other specialists. I tried every alternative treatment out there: acupuncture, THC, physical therapy, hypnosis, photomodulation, and neuromodulation (spinal cord stimulator), etc. The harder I tried to solve my pain and despair, the more I realized that my life had been permanently narrowed to a fraction of what it had been.

About five months ago, I went to see a new pain doctor in Charlotte, NC who suggested that I try LDN. I was completely open to the idea. I was told that it would take three months for me to see if it was going to help me. I am here to tell you that today, I am 95% pain-free. Instead of staying on the sofa, I am walking six and seven miles per day. I have done several destination walks of over 20 miles! I am on track to reach 1,000 miles walked by the end of June. This is astounding and I attribute every bit of my new pain free life to LDN!

One good thing that came out of this is that I started a positive support group for people with neuropathy. It's called Peripheral Neuropathy Success Stories. I just knew that people with this condition needed a positive place to find support. All of the other online support groups seemed so depressing and dire. I am so proud that this group is serving so many people in pain, in a positive way.

I am so happy to share my experience with LDN with everyone I know having pain. Dr. Leonardo Kapural, one of the top pain research doctors in the world, spoke to my neuropathy group about LDN earlier in the year. Since that time, I know many people who have started LDN and I am already hearing their successes.

My advice for anyone in pain is to try all available options. For me, LDN has been the very best option that I have tried.

Joyce, USA – Multiple Autoimmune Conditions

I am a 55-year-old female. I was first diagnosed with fibromyalgia in approximately 2017. Then I was diagnosed with Raynaud's disease, Graves' disease and Hashimoto's in 2019.

I developed hidradenitis suppurativa, then severe allergic response due to autoimmune issues. I have had osteoarthritis since the late 1990s, as well as GERD. My inflammation markers were through the roof. I was one marker away from lupus, and was tested for leukemia and MS due to my symptoms and repeated poor blood test results.

My doctors prescribed duloxetine, gabapentin, methimazole, famotidine, atorvastatin, mupirocin, allergy meds, doxycycline and many others along the way, trying to find something that would calm my autoimmune and thyroid issues.

My life was progressively becoming more difficult to manage. My pain levels, low energy, heart palpitations, weight gain, poor blood test results, and high inflammation had caused my work life to end. I was no longer able to manage household chores, a job, or even commuting to events outside the home due to poor health, depression and anxiety. At times, I would be bedridden, have weeks-long insomnia, or narcoleptic episodes, and many many other issues.

I eventually tried to get on disability after losing multiple jobs due to my health, which, even with help from a disability lawyer, I did not succeed at. I was at my lowest of lows, depressed, sick, at times immobile and thinking my life was over at 55.

Then, in early 2023, I saw a testimonial for LDN on a social media site. I thought it was too good to be true, another snake oil, out of my reach. I began researching every shred of information I could on this product. Then, armed with a head full of facts, figures and information, I timidly approached my doctor. I discussed what I had learned with her. She was familiar with it, and together we decided we had nothing more to lose, and everything to gain by trying LDN. We made arrangements and I began my LDN adventure.

I have been on 3 mg once daily for three months now. I started on a morning dose, but have recently, and more successfully, switched to evening dosage. I have regular blood tests and check-ups. My inflammation markers are reduced drastically. My cholesterol and blood sugar are back in the low normal range. My pain levels are reduced by about 80%. My sleep has greatly improved. My gut issues are greatly improved. I am no longer depressed or anxious. I have been taken off all my other prescription meds. My allergies cleared. My thyroid numbers normalized. I am no longer puffy and bloated. I am back to chasing grandkids and gardening, and have even taken on some babysitting to help my finances.

As for side effects, they were minimal. I experienced a red flushing and itching on the sites of my worst inflammation. I had sleepy spells after taking my LDN and a small but tolerable stomach issue. All these side effects remedied themselves within a few days.

I thank God for whoever discovered LDN. I have my life back. I am living again!

Jill Brook, USA – POTS, MCAS and Neuropathy

I was hanging by a thread when I discovered LDN. I'd had a 17-year diagnostic delay until my dozens of symptoms were diagnosed as POTS (postural orthostatic tachycardia syndrome), MCAS (mast cell activation syndrome) and autoimmune autonomic neuropathy.

My worst symptoms were fainting, major leg pain, a nightly stabbing itch, painful rashes, pressure-induced pain/swelling (meaning I couldn't get comfortable unless neck-deep in water), all sorts of allergies to foods/odors and even vibration (e.g., I went into anaphylaxis from riding over a bumpy road), ringing ears, hands that would puff up and burn at night and a lot of GI symptoms. Yes, I was a MESS!

It felt like such an accomplishment to endure these symptoms through a day, but then I'd remember that I still had to make it through the night, and I'd fall into despair. I'd tried all the many "normal" drugs for POTS and MCAS - taking 28 daily pills at one point - and some of them worked for a while, but then they'd wear off. In desperation I used a charity auction to buy a phone call with Dr. Pradeep Chopra, pain doctor extraordinaire. He suggested I try LDN.

That was eight years ago and WOW, is life ever better now. I took 4.5 mg and within a few days I felt different. I felt "psyched," like the feeling of a runner's high. My pain, energy, inflammation and sleep improved within a couple weeks. The only negative side effect was weird dreams, so I switched to morning dosing and that resolved. The positive side effect I felt was a reduced cravings for sweets, which helped me finally have the willpower to adopt a fully unprocessed diet.

Now I'm on three daily pills (LDN plus thyroid replacement). I have a happy life back again and my health isn't perfect, but it's good enough. LDN came along just in time for me. I'm not sure I was going to last much longer in my pre-LDN state.

I feel super lucky that LDN also appears to have some other health perks, unlike most drugs. I'm also grateful for the LDN Research Trust because I've learned it's a great way to discover physicians who are thought leaders and critical thinkers. Thanks, LDN Research Trust!

After hearing of my experience, several of my family members have tried LDN for joint pain/inflammation. One family member no longer needed a shoulder replacement, another was able to cancel her knee replacement (and she's hiking and snowshoeing again), and a third had his shoulder recover after years of PT that didn't help. Amazing!

Erica, UK – Multiple Autoimmune Conditions

I have suffered from MCAS for many years, with muscle and joint pain, interstitial cystitis pain, skin inflammation – particularly in my scalp, and a whole plethora of other unpleasant symptoms that made living a mere existence rather than a life. Things improved slightly when I had identified some of my triggers, and some of the medication, such as cimetidine and ketotifen, also helped a little but although the symptoms reduced somewhat, some were still troublesome.

In 2020 I also got COVID which was fairly mild really, but once it passed, I was left with an altered sense of smell – nothing smelled like it should have done or didn't smell of anything at all.

MCAS was of course my main concern and I searched online to find a better solution to what my immunologist was prescribing for me. After much reading it seemed that a lot of people with MCAS were talking favourably about one particular medication called low dose naltrexone.

I took some information to my immunologist and he basically ridiculed it and told me to continue with the things he had prescribed. Not being one to give in easily, being sick of being in pain and getting nowhere with doctors, I continued searching for a way to get this safe -sounding drug privately. That's when I found the LDN Research

Trust website with its list of prescribers and I was thankful to see that there was one in the UK.

I got my LDN medication five months ago and in that short time it has been life changing. By the end of week two on LDN my sense of smell returned to normal. By the end of the first month I felt more energetic and I realised that my inflammation, which just drained me physically, was much reduced. My scalp was clear after six weeks. The pain in my joints and muscles is also significantly reducing, as is my cystitis pain. I'm still in a state of disbelief really. I feel so much better and actually alive and hopeful for the future.

I didn't have any side effects whatsoever, perhaps because I increased slowly as my private doctor recommended. I take 3 mg at bedtime. I tried to increase to 3.5 mg but that didn't seem as good so I settled on 3 mg. I no longer take the other drugs now, just LDN and some supplements. I don't miss the other drugs at all.

I am so grateful for all the people on the internet who share their experiences, and all of the websites like the LDN Research Trust for raising awareness of this wonderful medication. I still avoid my triggers. I'm not going to make LDN's job harder than it needs to be but I'm happy, much more alive and I have hope for a full life without pain. I wish I'd known about this when I first became ill. It would have saved me many years of grief and pain. Thank you to everyone who strives to help others with otherwise untreatable illnesses.

Dianna, USA – Multiple Autoimmune Conditions

I had breast cancer in 2001 in my left breast. In 2006 it was in my right breast. In 2010 my left breast again. I had surgeries (lumpectomies each time) in 2001 in Newport News, Virginia (radiation follow up), in 2006 at Johns Hopkins, Maryland (follow up radiation and chemotherapy which wiped out my immune system) and in 2010 at Johns Hopkins Baltimore, Maryland (follow up radiation again).

My life was extremely difficult with cancers and other diagnoses, and extreme stress and depression.

After the third round with cancers in 2010 I learned about low dose naltrexone from the social media group "LDN GOT ENDORPHINS?

Low Dose Naltrexone" before I became one of the admins. I could not find a doctor to prescribe LDN. A member of the group had a list of doctors which she sent me and I contacted Dr. Coleman from Richmond, VA.

I had learned that I have Hashimoto's, Ehlers-Danlos type 3 (hypermobility), rheumatoid arthritis, fibromyalgia, and other autoimmune diseases and an extremely compromised immune system – a consequence of chemotherapy.

Dr. Coleman had previously only prescribed naltrexone as an opioid antagonist in much higher doses for use in alcohol disorders and opioid dependence. I called and asked Dr. Coleman if he would prescribe naltrexone for me in low doses. He had not heard of naltrexone in low doses to prevent cancers or for autoimmune conditions and asked if I could send him the information. I sent him the information that I had and after reading it he said he would see me and he prescribed LDN starting at 1.5 mg.

I stayed on that dose for months then went up to 2 mg. A few months later I tried 3 mg. I had negative results from 3 mg, extreme tailbone pain, left side felt weak, headache. I skipped the next dose and then went back to 2 mg. Months later I increased to 2 mg every 12 hours which seemed to be my perfect dose since I'm extremely sensitive to medications and could not tolerate 3 mg all at once.

It had taken me about three months to realize the benefits after first starting LDN.

The first LDN book came out and I ordered extra copies and gave copies to Dr. Peter Coleman and my PCP Dr. April Guminsky. After giving my PCP the LDN book she thanked me several times and she now prescribes LDN to other patients. My doctors also changed my diet, first AIP, then paleo, and now keto with no dairy.

Since taking LDN I've not had cancers – it's now April 2023. I tell others about LDN and direct them to the LDN Research Trust website and I post the information about LDN where I'm an Admin on social media on several groups.

At this time my Hashimoto's, RA, fibromyalgia diagnoses are currently in "remission" and "ALL" of my labs are excellent. LDN has made an AMAZING difference in my life and I feel that LDN has saved my life!

Yolanda, USA - Rheumatoid Arthritis and Hashimoto's

I was first diagnosed with Hashimoto's in October 2011, and a few months later with rheumatoid arthritis.

I was initially taking Synthroid for the Hashimoto's. For the RA, I was prescribed sulfasalazine for the entire time I saw the rheumatologist. I was also using Humira, methotrexate, Plaquenil, and taking folate for the methotrexate. So that's a total of five different medications taken at one time. But I had little to no improvement in my overall symptoms.

I spent approximately one year after I got diagnosed doing research. LDN kept popping up as I did research but a lot of the information came primarily from "Stop the Thyroid Madness."

It turned out that one of the naturopaths that I initially saw knew about LDN but she didn't prescribe it for nearly a year after I began to see her. She took credit for my having changed my diet and she had nothing to do with my decision to change my diet by eating AIP.

I started LDN at 0.5 mg and was given instructions to titrate up every few weeks until I got to 4.5 mg.

I primarily felt a difference with the RA. My pain level had gone down a lot. I could use my hands for work without worrying about the joints in my hands. The pain I had from the RA was in my right hand and foot. The RA kept getting better and better and I could tell the inflammation was leaving my body. I lost half a shoe size and all my shoes no longer fit. I had rings on my fingers that were constantly spinning on my hand since they were now too big.

LDN did help my RA but I have been told that it will work on the most serious illness/disease first. That's why I believe that it took so long for the RA to go fully into remission. Over the 12 years that I was taking LDN and seeing my rheumatologist, she would request MRIs, CAT scans, labs, to verify that the joints in my fingers were degenerative and she said I would end up with deformed hands like so many people with RA have. Three years ago my RA went into full remission, the joints in my hands seeming to regenerate. And to think my rheumatologist was annoyed with me for not wanting the mainstream drugs that did nothing for me.

For the Hashimoto's, the antibodies consistently kept going down until they're now at 14 and I'm essentially in remission with that. I had more problems with the RA than Hashimoto's. I have had two very painful surgeries but because of the LDN I was able to begin physical therapy with little to no problem. I love my LDN and want it to take care of all my issues.

Jennifer, Australia - Fibromyalgia and Osteoarthritis

I started using LDN about four years ago now. My life changed instantly from being in constant day and night chronic pain from fibromyalgia and osteoarthritis to being without pain!!

Before LDN I had been taking massive amounts of Panadol/ Naprosyn plus trying out many other types of medications to try to help cope with this illness. Despite those pain medications I still had pain.

I had heard of LDN so I bought the *The LDN Book* and managed to get myself a prescriber. Once I started LDN I then documented my progress in a journal daily. At the start I could hardly hold the pen to write. I ached day and night. I got so I didn't want to live, not in constant pain.

LDN gave me back my life. I can now live a normal life without pain. Thank you, Dr. Bihari, for saving my life!!!

Ania, Poland – Nerve Pain, Interstitial Cystitis and Arthritis

For nine years I suffered with nerve pain, interstitial cystitis and general arthritis pain. From 2009 to 2018 I was prescribed morphine sulphate twice a day and other OTC painkillers to supplement the morphine. I had periodic lumbar epidural steroid injections which did help. I was also taking Ambien to help me sleep and Xanax for my anxiety – something that comes with constant pain unfortunately. The morphine helped with the pain but it doesn't provide what might be called "a life" – I was sleepy all the time, couldn't really think properly and it made me slightly nauseous. It also gave me constipation so I had to take laxatives.

I had built a pretty strong tolerance for opiates and it was decided, late in 2018, that it was time to wean off it. This took a long time and wasn't pleasant.

Around 2019 I got a new doctor and he talked to me about LDN. He said it would help me wean off the opiates, which wouldn't be so bad, he said, because I'd already started that detoxing process. I started LDN on very small microgram doses and increased the LDN as I reduced the morphine. I had to be under close supervision by my doctors while I was reducing the morphine, especially once the LDN was added, as the withdrawal can be horrible, though I didn't really have too much trouble after the LDN was started. The pain I had to begin with was bad too but I persevered. Being permanently drugged is no way to live.

As the LDN dose increased and the morphine use was minimal my pain started to get much better. I think overall it took about six months to be completely off the morphine. It seemed to go quicker once the LDN was added. Since mid-2019 I no longer needed morphine, I'm much more energetic and my head is clear and I feel that I want to live again. I'd lost the will to live over all those years of constant pain. It was just endless misery. I no longer need laxatives as the morphine has gone and I'm off Xanax and Ambien too.

I have no nerve, arthritis or cystitis pain now. I have my life back and want to live it. LDN has been a godsend to me. It feels like a miracle. I know it isn't a cure. I have to keep taking it to maintain the wonderful benefits but that's fine because there is nothing negative about LDN. I didn't experience any horrible side effects to speak of. I'm astounded that LDN is not offered routinely for pain issues rather than opiates. I wish my doctors had offered me it sooner and I'm actually quite angry that they didn't.

Laurie, USA – Multiple Autoimmune Conditions

My name is Laurie. I live in Missouri where I own and operate a bed and breakfast. I have been taking low dose naltrexone for approximately 13 years.

I have been sick for most of my life. I actually have 17 different diagnoses that I am living with. I have osteo, rheumatoid and psoriatic arthritis, fibromyalgia, degenerative disc disease, MCTD, MGUS, lupus, Raynaud's, systemic scleroderma, bronchiectasis, myasthenia gravis, interstitial lung disease, lymphoma, hemolytic anemia, and hypergammaglobulinemia. I was prescribed traditional medicines for most of my life and I was only declining. I was unable to dress or walk without assistance. My pain was very real. My quality of life was not good at all.

I was desperate to find a treatment that would work for me. I had a friend, who had been on LDN for several years, who encouraged me to ask my doctor about it. I was the first patient that my doctor had given LDN to. She had read about it and felt that it was very safe and was confident that I couldn't get any worse from trying it. We both decided to begin the process to see if it would help me. I had no idea what to expect. I had gotten my hopes up many times with other medications only to be let down.

I had been on LDN for a few months when I woke up one morning and I had no pain. At first, I thought that it was just odd and it probably wouldn't happen again. But it did! Several days passed and I was still pain free. I had strength to dress and walk without assistance. I was able to do things that I had not done in years. It gave me a new life!

Many things have happened since the beginning. The diseases that I have been diagnosed with are progressive. I have had a few setbacks but my doctors are beyond amazed at how I bounce back each time!! In fact, a few years back, I was diagnosed with respiratory failure and I was prescribed supplemental oxygen 24/7. I was not expected to recover but I did. I was able to get off of the oxygen and I not only survived but I am thriving.

Despite the diagnoses that I have been given, low dose naltrexone has given me an excellent quality of life! I am pain free and I don't even look sick. I am able to travel with my family and own and operate a successful business. I never could have imagined this before low dose naltrexone.

Jackie, USA - Ehlers-Danlos Syndrome and Crohn's Disease

I first got sick with Crohn's disease right before my 29th birthday. I ended up needing emergency surgery four months after my first Crohn's symptoms appeared. I had a total of eight surgeries in a two-year time period. I had complication after complication. We now know that my complications are because of a rare genetic condition that affects my connective tissue called Ehlers-Danlos syndrome, which I was diagnosed with at 35 years old.

I was given many doses of different IV antibiotics called fluroquinolones (which are known to destroy connective tissue). That is when my pain started.

I lived at a ten on the pain scale for a very long time. My kids weren't even able to hug me because every touch felt excruciatingly painful. I was miserable! My entire body felt like I had gotten hit by a bus all the time. I was beyond exhausted. People with EDS tend to get "painsomnia." I wasn't sleeping very much because I was in so much pain.

I first heard about LDN from my allergist, Dr. Ariana Buchanan in Carrollton, GA. She suggested that I ask my GP about trying it. Thankfully, my GP, Dr. Megan Bowles, was familiar with the use of LDN for people like me. She wrote me a script for 1.5 mg that day (which is the same dose I'm still taking now), and I took my first pill that evening. That night was the first night in YEARS that I actually got deep sleep, and woke up feeling rested. The following day, I had an extra boost of energy from all of the extra endorphins, that I haven't felt in many years. I actually cried that day because that was the first glimpse of hope that I had in quite a while.

Before LDN, I had given up all hope of ever having a decent quality of life. That "hit by a bus" feeling now only comes towards the end of the day, or if I overdo it. Thankfully, I didn't have any lasting side effects when I started taking LDN. I did have an increase in anxiety for only one week. LDN has significantly decreased my pain level. I also have noticed an improvement in my brain fog.

I tell everyone I know with a chronic illness about it because it has helped me so immensely. It has been a game changer for me! Everyone around me can see the improvements in me. Thankfully I was one of the lucky ones who got immediate results from this medication. Do I still have pain and struggles? Yes, absolutely, but they are way more manageable since starting LDN. I'm hopeful once I get to the full dose of 4.5 mg, I will feel even better.

Lena, Denmark – Multiple Autoimmune Conditions

I am 46 years old and I suffer from osteoarthritis, chronic nerve pain, Modic changes, muscle pain and I have a herniated disc in my back. My symptoms started in 2008 and due to the pain my social life became very limited.

I could not do the same tasks at home or work as I used to and I was often on sick leave from work. I tried various pain killers such as morphine and nerve medication without optimal effect. Doing my own research, I found a social media group dedicated to chronic pain and that's where I first heard about LDN.

I had to go to a pain clinic to get LDN prescribed. Initially I was on too high a dose for me, 2.25 mg, and I had side effects so I reduced my dose to 0.125 mg, and after a few days the side effects disappeared. After a few weeks on this dose I started to feel benefits and six months later was 100% pain free.

This was seven years ago and I was able to keep my job and do all the things I should be able to do, with no pain. I would definitely recommend that others who suffer chronic pain at least try LDN. For me it's been a life changer.

Susan, UK - Myalgic Encephalomyelitis and Fibromyalgia

I was diagnosed with fibromyalgia in 1997 then ME in 1998, having suffered with fluctuating symptoms since my early teens (1982 onwards). I then heard about LDN in 2014. I was in the moderate to severely affected group with my symptoms, housebound 24/7 with most days bedbound.

I had also been diagnosed early 2014 with antiphospholipid syndrome and possible mild lupus, other autoimmune conditions and my inflammatory markers were very high.

I came across the LDN Research Trust on social media and read up on all their literature, and other patients' success stories. I decided it was something I would like to try so I downloaded the information sheets from LDN Research Trust's website and showed it to my GP. To my surprise my GP agreed to write me a private prescription to try it as all other treatments and medications I'd tried over the years for my ME either proved to be of no benefit or gave me too many unpleasant side effects.

I started on 1.5 mg of the liquid LDN which I obtained from a pharmacy in Glasgow. I had no adverse effects and increased it after a few weeks to 2 mg, then 2.5 mg a few weeks later, continuing every few weeks to 4 mg but found that too much, making my ME symptoms worse again so I ended up finding a comfortable baseline of 3 mg.

My inflammatory markers six months later were all normal and I started to notice I could do more before being hit with the usual debilitating fatigue and the ensuing PEM. My brain fog lifting was one of the first things I noticed about six weeks after I started on it. I have stayed on 3 mg for over eight years now but have just recently successfully upped it to 3.5 mg.

So how has it improved my quality of life? Let's just say I notice the difference when I don't take it. I ran out over Christmas due to postal strikes and was off it for three weeks, resulting in a huge flare and eventually being confined to my bed again every day. But after a few weeks back on it I started to feel much better again. All my inflammatory markers had begun to creep up over the normal range on my blood tests but they soon went back to normal a few weeks after being back on my daily dose of LDN.

It hasn't cured my ME as I still have to pace every day, not do too many activities without resting and be mindful not to push my body beyond its limits in order to avoid crashing, but it gives me a life worth living.

Jacqui, Australia – Multiple Autoimmune Conditions

My main reason for wanting to try LDN was for my consistently high level of chronic pain which averaged a 6-9 daily on a pain scale for over six years and 24 hours a day. I can't take opioids so I needed something gentle enough with low side effects if any at all and no withdrawal.

The other main reason I wanted to try LDN was for my consistently-high inflammation markers shown in my CRP and ESR blood tests (and systemic inflammation shown in my lumbar puncture test).

Lastly, I hoped for immune modulation as I have a long history of infections and subsequent diseases, including dengue fever, Q fever and various tick-borne diseases including Lyme; and I had read it's also good for MCAS mast cell stabilisation.

I first noticed my chronic health symptoms in 2017. They were moderate to extreme symptoms when my Lyme and co-infections showed up in tests and symptoms after an extreme physical exertion and dental surgery, and also it was two months after a tick bite. However, I have had a lifetime of various illnesses and diseases/infections.

My life has been extremely difficult over the last seven years - the normal Lyme, fibro and CFS/ME symptoms plus my chronic pain was debilitating. I also suffered syncope often and back-to-back seizures and was predominantly bed bound each and every day for approximately 80-90% of day. I was unable to work or drive a car anymore and suffered the loss of independence.

I've tried multiple Lyme treatments in Australia, and abroad. They include antibiotics, supplements, diet changes and juices, acupuncture, lifestyle changes, and ozone therapy etc. I wasn't on any medication for pain or immune modulation.

Accessing LDN was really difficult in Australia. I first read about it in 2017 and I had asked over six doctors in four to five years for a trial of LDN until I finally found one committed to trialling me on it. Now I am on a dose of 6 mg per day, but I have met with resistance to trial a higher dose for residual pain, or to try two doses per day, but grateful to have access finally to LDN.

I started LDN in 2021 on 1.5 mg as an initial dose but it was too high. After a short break the doctor agreed on a lower dose of 0.5 mg for me to start with and it suited me much better (MCAS makes me more sensitive than most to new drugs and I can get anaphylaxis or reactions to new drugs). I took it low and slow for LDN - 0.5 start and only increased by 0.5 every four to six weeks. It took approximately 11 months to get to 4.5 mg and only then did I feel the larger more noticeable benefits.

My dose is now 6 mg and it suits me better than 4.5. I'm not pain free but it has knocked down my pain significantly and I'm delighted to say it's shifted my inflammation markers to finally within range for the first time in over six years! Nothing else has even moved the inflammation including antibiotics treatment and ozone etc., nor special anti-inflammation juices and special diets.

On an initial dose of 1.5 mg I suffered a flare in my pain and also my "brain on fire," migraines with auras and head pressure. I lasted only one to two weeks trying to push through and then took a break and restarted at 0.5 as mentioned. I have since discovered I have severe internal jugular vein compression (two sub types of Eagle syndrome), plus white matter lesions and considerable calcification in the brain, so perhaps this contributed to my inability to go too fast/high on LDN ?

Going forward with LDN titration, the only time I had side effects was when I increased my dose by 0.5 mg but at this small increase it was usually mild to moderate only in intensity, and usually body or head pain or both and it would dissipate within a week or even a few days. It was bearable and temporary. If side effects hung around longer, I knew I wasn't ready for a higher dose yet and stayed at the lower dose for longer before trying again.

My most noticeable improvements as mentioned above took 11 months. When I finally reached a dose of 4.5 mg, that's when I noticed less pain every day and my ability to push myself a little more in day to day tasks and with lower payback or post-exertional malaise. However prior to that point I did note a small change in my pain levels but only when I accidentally ran out of my script and had to go a week off LDN - that timeframe off LDN told me that LDN benefits can be very subtle improvements, so much so that you can miss them entirely.

For transparency I currently take about four to five scripted medications (mainly MCAS mix and an anti-epilepsy med), plus a few supplements like vitamin C, D and magnesium.

LDN is without a doubt THE best drug I have added to my list of medications. As someone that has lived a torture of ongoing pain 24-7 for over six years at extreme levels - any respite from this is so remarkable and welcome. Sure, I'm not pain free and I can still get pain flares if I overdo it but I think if you have real expectations for what it can do for you then most will be pleasantly surprised. I also love the fact there is no withdrawal on this drug for if I need surgery etc.

I guess for me I would love to know if LDN is helping to repair what caused my inflammation or is it very possible if I come off it one day will it all return? I know treating the cause is important, which is highly likely infection and Lyme related, but I'm curious about research on LDN and inflammation.

Also I'm terrified of losing another doctor in my country and not being able to source more LDN. I would love you to talk to our health department, and/or pain clinics etc., to ask them to recognise the benefit of LDN and get the word out there. It's a miracle drug.

PETS

Francie, USA – Dogs, Horses and a Cat

Since taking LDN for my MS and having great results, and since my husband, Chuck's, great results with LDN for his allergies, we started to use LDN for our dogs, horses and my mother's cat. We run a big ranch so have lots of animals. I'd done my research and found so many success stories about LDN and pets so wasn't particularly worried that anything bad would happen.

We started by giving the LDN to my mother's ancient cat. I swear that it bought her an extra nine lives. My mom could not dose the kitty herself, so the cat only got LDN about two or three times per week when somebody else was there to administer it. This is where we learned that "pulse" dosing (every couple of days) also does work, and that some LDN is better than none.

I want to list just some of the disorders in animals that we have used it for over the years:

Rain rot. This is a fungal attack that can come with the change in weather and lowered immune system. We had three Friesian colts that we weaned at the same time that the weather changed and all three got rain rot. The vet wanted us to bathe them with an antibacterial soap daily for a week. But it was cold and these colts were not savvy about holding still to have cold water sprayed on them, so we put each of them on 5 mg of LDN. Within three days, the rain rot was already clearing up. We use 5 mg for young horses or Caspian horses of about 500 pounds and 6 mg for larger 1,000 to 1,200 pound horses. We believe that the dose is related to the number of receptor sites, not so much the weight of the horse.

Allergies in dogs. This is especially useful for flea allergies and food allergies. It can take a bit for the LDN to kick in and eliminate the allergies, but the dog can be on other treatments at the same time to bridge the gap. The dose is 0.03 mg per pound, so a 33-pound dog gets 1 mg and a 50 pound dog gets 1.5 mg, for instance.

I am not sure if it made a difference, but we had an outbreak of parvo in our puppies last year and lost three straight litters. There was a fourth litter, younger and still probably protected by the mother's antibodies. But we put the baby puppies on LDN and then administered ½ of a parvo vaccination each week. Two of them showed symptoms, but none of them died. We feel that the improved immune system and vigilance made the difference in helping these babies to survive.

We have two white horses that are brothers, two years apart at 33 and 35 years old. One has cancer of the sheath, but we have held off a crisis for years now with the use of LDN.

LDN does not make one immortal, but can help a person or pet live a healthy life until the day that they die. Avoiding the long slow decline in health at the advanced age is priceless.

We don't use LDN on all horses or all dogs, all the time. We really have too many for that, but we do use it any time that we feel that the immune system needs a boost, or if there is advanced age.

Kody and Paula, UK – Canine Arthritis

Kody is a female Alaskan Malamute x German Shepherd cross, a very large dog. When Kody was only four years old she started limping badly on her right front paw. The vet said it was arthritis. Front leg arthritis is horrible, especially when the dog wants to be upstairs. Them coming down scares the hell out of me. Kody was pretty bad, especially after a chase of something, she would be struggling for days and then settle back to a manageable limp but I could see it was hurting her, and having arthritis myself I understand that pain.

I didn't want to put her on the drugs the vet was offering as they tend to mess up the liver and with her only being four I thought she was too young to start on such as Rimadyl – not so bad when they're older perhaps but not at four.

I realised that it was likely autoimmune. Why would she have arthritis at that age? I put her on LDN after a lot of reading about other people's experiences with their pets. Naltrexone, in low doses, is non-toxic and the side effects are minimal and transitory. I read a lot of testimonials from people who had given LDN to their cats, dogs, horses and they were all really positive. I couldn't find any negatives.

Kody's arthritis resolved in three days and after three months I thought that maybe I could take her off it, maybe it had been an injury? So I took her off it and three days later she's limping again. I put her back on it, just 2 mg at night, and she was fine in three days and hasn't limped since and Kody is 12 in October and is doing really well.

Fiona and Dana, USA – Canine IBS

My 6-year-old mastiff named Fiona was suffering from IBS. She wasn't eating food several times during the week and had bloody stool. The first vet I took her to only gave her antibiotics. This did not improve her health.

Since I was taking LDN for Crohn's disease I sought out a vet, about one hour away, who would write out a prescription for LDN for her. We also took her off kibble and started cooking her turkey, beef, fish and vegetables.

We started her on 2 mg capsules of LDN and increased it to 2.5 and then eventually 3 mg. She took this for five years and it greatly improved her health. She rarely missed a meal and no longer suffered from diarrhea.

She did not experience any negative side effects from LDN at all. I have shared this valuable treatment information with others who have pets who suffer from IBS or IBD.

We believe that the LDN, along with a healthier diet, made such a difference to the quality of her life and hope that more animals will benefit as their owners learn about this reasonably priced, safe and highly effective treatment.

Basse and Anette, Denmark – Canine Bladder Cancer

On 18 May 2020, my 8-year-old dog Basse was diagnosed with bladder cancer when we had observed blood in his urine. The vet said that after a diagnosis of bladder cancer, dogs live a maximum of four months without treatment and 11 months with treatment such as meloxicam or chemotherapy.

The vet did not know about LDN but wanted to read up on it, and until the start of LDN (four days later) Basse was given meloxicam due to pain during urination.

Basse started LDN on 22 May 2020. He weighed 29 kg and therefore was given a dose of 2.9 mg daily. This seemed to make him a very tired dog for two days, so we reduced the dose to 2.4 mg and Basse was himself again.

On June 18th 2020, a urine sample check showed no blood and fewer cancer cells. Basse slept very well at night and no longer had to pee four or five times every night. Energy, activity level and appetite were really good.

27th July a check of his urine sample now showed only a few cancer cells left.

On September 18th, a urine sample check showed very few cancer cells left and they are no longer aggressive and do not divide.

A year after the diagnosis, a check of the urine showed that there are absolutely no cancer cells left.

Basse lived cancer-free until he was euthanized in August 2022 due to severe dementia. He lived to be 10.5 years old and neither of his parents or siblings lived more than 8-9 years, so he did well and had a good life.

Sil and Aure, Amsterdam – Feline Intestinal Lymphoma

My friend's cat Sil was diagnosed with lymphoma (intestinal) stage 4 in August of 2019. He was given prednisolone and just three months to live. Right after the colonoscopy, the vet put him on 5 mg prednisone. Sil (male) had just turned 13 and he was clearly feeling unwell. He was less social, not eating well, easily startled, not going out on the balcony as he used to do.

I told my friend about LDN and that it could work well for cancer. So we talked to her vet, contacted Skip's pharmacy in Florida to confirm the right dose for a cat, and started Sil on LDN.

His first dose was about two weeks after his diagnosis. Sil became a bit more wobbly at first, but three or four days later my friend saw a big change. He started eating normally again, going outside, became his own social, cuddly, goofy self again. He clearly had more energy again and his stools also improved. He had been doing well on 0.3 mg LDN and 5 mg prednisone for almost four years.

In September 2022 he started losing weight, became a bit restless and very picky with food. Blood tests showed low B12 and hyperthyroidism. Slowly he lost more weight. He was clearly going downhill, but most likely due to old age. A couple of weeks ago he had a stroke, followed by a second one last Friday. My friend made the heartbreaking decision to have him put to sleep. However sad it was, LDN has given them almost four more years of good quality life together and that was priceless to both of them!

Roxy and Toby, Australia – Canine Cushing's Disease

I rescued Roxy, my dog, at age 11. She was starved. She soon gained weight but became puffy. The vet diagnosed Cushing's disease and prescribed trilostane tablets. The vet said that dogs never heal from Cushing's and it would only be helped with trilostane which she would be on for the rest of her life. Roxy's blood was taken every three months and the trilostane dose was adjusted accordingly. Roxy was ill when I rescued her so I can only assume she felt dreadful for a long period of time given the starvation and the diagnosis from the vet.

I first heard about LDN from my niece who suffers with lupus. She told me about it when I was diagnosed with scleroderma. I have taken LDN myself for years so, after reading up on pets and LDN, I decided to try LDN for Roxy at a dose of 1.2 mg as per her weight.

My local vet refused to prescribe LDN for Roxy so I searched the internet and I found and contacted The Healing Vet on social media. He had never used LDN but was willing to write a script and follow Roxy's progress via phone. This was in 2018.

Roxy started on 1.2 mg and remained on that dose throughout the rest of her life. I noted no side effects whatsoever but within three months it was noted by the vet that Roxy needed a reduction in her dose of trilostane – this was unusual according to the vet. Within the year her blood work showed that trilostane was no longer needed. Since the vet said healing from Cushing's was unheard of, I assume it was the LDN that healed her.

LDN gave Roxy four more healthy years, which was wonderful for both of us. She was almost 16 when she died. I did keep her on LDN even after her Cushing's disease had disappeared.

I still take LDN and it allows me to live a full and (mostly) pain free life.

A Study on the use of LDN as a Chemotherapy Adjuvant for Dogs

The objective of this study was to evaluate the effect of low dose naltrexone (LDN) as a chemotherapy-adjuvant in female dogs with mammary carcinoma in benign mixed tumors (MC-BMT) after mastectomy and to assess its association with quality of life and survival rates.

The conclusion of this study states that the results demonstrate that naltrexone reduces the side effects related to carboplatin chemotherapy. Naltrexone treatment increased beta-endorphin and met-enkephalin serum concentrations, improved the animals' well-being, maintained their quality of life, and contributed to an increased survival rate in dogs undergoing chemotherapy, thus making LDN adjuvant treatment an important tool in the clinical management of mammary tumors in female dogs.

Machado, M. C. et al. (2018). The effect of naltrexone as a carboplatin chemotherapy-associated Drug on the immune response, quality of life and survival of dogs with mammary carcinoma. PloS one, 13(10).

–

EPILOGUE

The LDN Research Trust was established in 2004 by Linda Elsegood as a non-profit charity dedicated to raising awareness of low dose naltrexone (LDN), which has shown promising results in treating various autoimmune diseases, chronic pain, and other conditions. The charity provides information and support to patients interested in trying LDN as a treatment option and medical professionals who wish to learn more.

The LDN Research Trust collaborates with healthcare professionals, researchers, and patients worldwide to increase awareness and understanding of LDN and its potential benefits. They have a jam-packed website with over 2.6 million visitors a year.

The trust provides a wealth of information on LDN, including its benefits and uses through various platforms such as iTunes, Spotify, YouTube, Vimeo, Facebook Channels, etc. The trust also organizes monthly webinars and weekly radio shows and has published *The LDN Book* volumes 1, 2, and 3, which are widely used by medical professionals when prescribing and compounding LDN. Additionally, the trust has produced seven documentaries, with the last one released in June 2024. They have a closed Facebook group and Facebook pages, LinkedIn, X (formally Twitter) Health Unlocked and Pinterest.

The LDN Research Trust is celebrating its 20th anniversary this year. It has made remarkable achievements with the help of its dedicated volunteers, medical advisors, and speakers who work tirelessly to offer help and support as required. They rely on donations and medical memberships as they receive no funding. This financial support is crucial for the trust to continue its work.

ACKNOWLEDGMENTS

We extend our sincere gratitude to all the contributors who generously shared their LDN experiences and helped us celebrate our 20th anniversary. It is an honour to have so many amazing people taking part.

We would like to extend a special thanks to Paula Johnson for her hard work in editing and typesetting the book.

Lastly, but certainly not least, we would like to thank you, the reader, for your interest and support.

ABOUT THE EDITOR

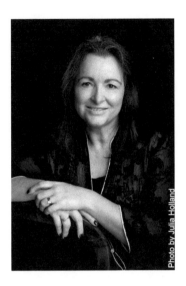

Linda Elsegood is the founder of the UK charity LDN Research Trust, established in 2004. She has Multiple Sclerosis (MS), and low dose naltrexone (LDN) has significantly impacted her life.

She wanted to help other people, not only with MS but with all autoimmune diseases, cancers, mental health issues, etc.

In the last 20 years, the charity has helped over a million people worldwide.